Brain Injury Rewiring

for Loved Ones

AN IDYLL ARBOR PERSONAL HEALTH BOOK

Brain Injury Rewiring

for Loved Ones

A Lifeline to New Connections

Carolyn E. Dolen, MA

Foreword by Nathan D. Zasler, MD

Idyll Arbor

Idyll Arbor, Inc.

39129 264th Ave SE, Enumclaw, WA 98022 (360) 825-7797

Idyll Arbor, Inc. Editor: Thomas M. Blaschko

Back cover photograph: Don Anderson

To the best of our knowledge, the information and recommendations of this book reflect currently accepted practice. Nevertheless, they cannot be considered absolute and universal. Recommendations for a particular person must be considered in light of the person's needs and condition. The author and publisher disclaim responsibility for any adverse effects resulting directly or indirectly from the suggested therapy practices, from any undetected errors, or from the reader's misunderstanding of the text.

18.05 **Library of Congress Cataloging-in-Publication Data**

Dolen, Carolyn E., 1946-
  Brain injury rewiring for loved ones : a lifeline to new connections / Carolyn E. Dolen ; foreword by Nathan D. Zasler.
      p. cm.
  "An Idyll Arbor Personal Health Book."
  Includes bibliographical references and index.
  ISBN 978-1-882883-71-4 (alk. paper)
  1. Brain damage--Patients--Family relationships. 2. Brain damage--Patients--Rehabilitation. 3. Caregivers. I. Title.
  RC387.5.D647 2010
  617.4'810443--dc22

                                                                    2009021782

ISBN 9781882883714

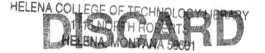

To all loved ones

That you see the sun
As well as the clouds.

That others share your journey
And lighten your load.

That you find what you seek.

And that by helping your survivor
You help yourself

To angels everywhere

Thank you for demonstrating that
"No act of kindness,
however small,
is ever wasted."
(Aesop)

Contents

Foreword

Brain injury can often be a major, life-changing event, not only for the person with the injury but also for family members and significant others. Clearly, at times, brain injury can be catastrophic, even to the point of ending life, either literally or at least as the person and their family knew it. Ultimately, recovering from such an injury can be a journey in and of itself. A journey that can often hold disappointment, as well as surprises, anxiety, frustration, anger and, yes, even joy. A journey that often is marked by doubt, questioning, and uncertainty.

Often times, families grapple with changes that they see in their injured loved one. They may look the same, but the "old person" may never actually be back... sometimes a very difficult thing to accept. The injured person may have died in a figurative sense, yet there was never a funeral or any other formal acknowledgement that the injured person is not the same. Families often need to get to know and love the "new" person... even if they are very different (and yet the same).

There are frequently questions of what should be done to optimize recovery or what types of activities should be avoided and, unfortunately and all too frequently, no good place to get the answers to these important questions.

Brain injury advice often is challenging due to the fact that no two brain injuries are alike, as well as the phenomena of brain injury being a spectrum disorder, that is, it can be mild to severe to everything in between. Mild TBI may impact function adversely on multiple levels including negatively effecting concentration, attention, executive skills such as prioritization abilities and organizational skills, producing affective or emotional lability and irritability, causing sleep difficulties, and producing symptoms of fatigue, headache, and dizziness, to name just a few. Moderate to severe TBI can produce prominent cognitive, behavioral, language, and physical impairments that dramatically impact the life of the affected person and also the lives of all who care for that person.

A family that has to deal with a loved one who is brain injured needs as much assistance as they can get their hands on. Having an understanding of how brain injury may change an individual's ability to function at home, in the workplace, and in community is critical to being able to deal with the alterations in function that may be observed following an acquired brain injury. Additionally, being educated as to what one can do to help the injured person adapt to their impairments, improve their functional independence, and "recover" is key to feeling empowered and effectuating change in both their life and that of their loved one.

In providing knowledge to family members, one not only empowers these individuals but also decreases the anxieties associated with the unknown and facilitates a more optimistic outlook on the future by explaining how family members can aid the recovery process of an injured loved one. Knowledge is power and I believe that such power also imbues a resiliency to the common stressors of dealing with significant disability in a loved one, including minimizing the chances of burnout.

All too often, in this age of modern medicine and "managed care," clinicians are disinclined to take the time to adequately educate families about the recovery process and what they can do to both optimize and contribute to it. The pressures of modern day medical practice, and professional practice in general, often limit the amount of time that family members of survivors get for education and training about what is truly required to not only understand the level of their loved one's brain injury but also become prepared to help them adequately deal with it in the context of their ongoing recovery and rehabilitation whether in the hospital or community.

Brain Injury Rewiring for Loved Ones: A Lifeline to New Connections by Carolyn Dolen is one part of a two-part series to assist persons with brain injury as well as their families in the recovery journey and should serve as an important resource regardless of the severity of the brain injury incurred. Ms. Dolen's book for loved ones parallels the book for survivors in terms of general content and approach. *Brain Injury Rewiring for Loved Ones* provides family members a comprehensive overview of brain injury, recovery, post-injury adaptation, and "life rehabilitation," in a way that is educational, readable, and relevant. Readers will find the admixture of science and practical recommendations refreshing.

The book begins nicely with a foundation relative to Ms. Dolen's brain injury experience and her perspectives garnered over the years of her recovery and adaptation. She then explores basic issues about brain anatomy, injury, recovery, and treatment that should be welcomed by all facing such issues given its scope and lay clarity. Ms. Dolen then carefully dissects various aspects of what is truly the multidimensionality of recovery, acceptance, and life success over the ensuing eight chapters and covers diverse topics such as spirituality, cognition, emotions, body-mind interactions, nutrition, physical aspects of injury and recovery, socializations issues, and return to work challenges.

The insertion of quotes throughout the text also adds to the multidimensionality of the information provided and will be refreshing for readers who may otherwise become overly focused on the serious matters at hand. The section on "resources," is wonderful and provides a unique and comprehensive listing of a diverse number of valuable organizations, resources, and websites that can serve as additional sources of information for families and significant others. Lastly, the references are listed in a very user-friendly manner by being divided by chapter and listed alphabetically by first author.

Ms. Dolen's journey and lessons learned as reflected in *Brain Injury Rewiring for Loved Ones* provides a unique perspective on one person's recovery after brain injury and, in that context, provides hope to others of their own ability to both understand and assist an injured loved one to recover control of their life following acquired brain injury. I know readers will find Ms. Dolen's *Brain Injury Rewiring for Loved Ones* an important educational and coping resource. If there ever was a "lifeline" for families after brain injury this is it.

Nathan D. Zasler, MD, FAAPM&R, FACRM, FAADEP, DAAPM, CBIST
CEO & Medical Director, Tree of Life Services, Inc.
CEO & Medical Director, Concussion Care Centre of Virginia, Ltd.
Consultant in Neurorehabilitation, NorthEast Center for Special Care

Acknowledgements

To rewire body, mind, and spirit after a brain injury requires lots of helpers (as described in Chapter Two). Here I will endeavor to thank all of the many angels whom God sent to me. More than thirty years have elapsed since I started this journey, and someone may be inadvertently omitted, despite God's efforts to awaken me at 5 AM with names on the brain! Please forgive me if I miss one of you. You all really did help, and survivors sometimes don't remember everything, as most of you undoubtedly already know.

This list starts with my best friend since 1976, Marlys Henke, who offered her hearth, as well as her heart, mind, and pocketbook many times during the course of our cross-country friendship. It all began with a chance encounter on our first day of teachers' meetings at Highland Park Junior High in St. Paul, Minnesota. I asked her to join several of us at lunch. Funny how it's all worked out. She invited me to her Methodist Church home, affiliated with United Ministries in Higher Education (UMHE), located on the University of Minnesota campus. This church connection also enriched our friendship. Indeed, God works in mysterious ways.

Another angel was my childhood friend, Louise Lentz, who nourished me and visited me, even in locked wards and other undesirable places, just because I needed her. Friends from Johnson High School, like Mike Kluznik, and St. Olaf College alum Ann Jorstad stuck with me through many travails and helped me to remember that I was still lovable and fun. So did Pat Marshall, a dear friend since the 1980s from my San Diego days.

"Body and spirit" professionals who were especially helpful fit into the "Friends" category because the best ones acted as professionals who were friends. My willpower alone would not have gotten me up the rehab mountain. I needed the loving persistence — and wisdom — of these special people, who believed, respected, and cared.

The first of these is DJ (Dale Johnson, PhD of El Paso, Texas), who unfortunately is not physically alive to see my current status on the mountain, but I know that he knows where I am. Without DJ, I'd probably still be kicking holes in desks, punching holes in walls, screaming, crying, and cutting and burning my arm — or in some state mental hospital, homeless, or dead. Until his death in 1991, DJ visited, called, and wrote to ensure my psyche stayed on course.

Significant professionals in the 1980s include Liana Beckett, an MFCC intern at the UCSD Gifford Clinic, who continued to help me sort out the puzzle, and Mary-Alice Isenhart, PhD, who taught me that it is okay to be a strong woman. My 1990s team starts with Christine Baser, PhD, who lovingly empowered me to make significant changes in a short amount of time. Dr. Baser referred me to Daniel Gardner, MD, who treated me with respect, which enabled me to trust a male psychiatrist, even with a nineteen-year history of failure, with both MDs and drugs. Another Dr. Baser referral, Kent Bennington, PhD, used Eye Movement Desensitization and Reprocessing (EMDR), to end my irrational fears relative to the trauma of a post-injury sexual assault in 1976 and the various associated fears from the auto accident that necessitated this long climb.

Nathan Zasler, MD, most assuredly belongs on this list, not only for his brain injury treatment guidance, suggesting the Brain Tuner that replaced Prozac, but also the faithful mentoring that began in January, 1995. Dr Z (as I call him) provided the first review of *Brain Injury Rewiring*, a critique that led to my first contract. Survivors everywhere thank you, Dr. Zasler, for igniting *Brain Injury Rewiring*!

While I've needed less care since 1999, angels who helped heal wounds included Margaret November, MD, who noticed my occasional twitching, heretofore unrecognized, and prescribed Neurontin, which I can also use if/when I feel depressed or anxious. (The grey and cold winters still plague me.) Then in 2008 when I experienced PTSD from two rear-end collisions in a year, I sought an EMDR practitioner because it worked so well previously. Fortunately, I found my current on-call angel, Kay Emerick, PhD, with whom I immediately connected. She, like the other best helpers, maintained eye contact, took few notes, and seemed to actually like me — even expressing it! Other current loving members of my health care team include acupuncturist Mike Long, chiropractor Robert Cocain, DC, and Gulnar Poorsattar, MD. I feel very blessed!

To heal my spirit, I looked to the church, which lightened my load on many occasions. Early on, in 1976-78, it was Bill Mate, minister at UMHE, who patiently provided weekly counseling when no other services could or would handle my morass of problems. As part of the University outreach program, Bill, a noted writer, led a weekly group on writing exercises that ventured into safe areas and provided a wonderful escape route for me.

Following Bill in 1978 was a minister in El Paso, Texas. She and her family took me in after the YWCA called with a desperate plea for housing for a woman with a disabled vehicle, who was far from home — and without funds. This kind family offered a sanctuary for me for several weeks, and the Catholic Church accepted me in worship, even without nice clothes. Another early angel was the tow truck driver in Van Horn, Texas, who invited me to stay with him and his other three roommates (without disturbing me!) because I had no money and no place to go after the engine of my MG blew up in the Van Horn Mountains on my way from Minnesota to California in 1980. Thank you, too, for towing my MG to El Paso out of the goodness of your heart.

During my El Paso stay, a call from a friend brought me to New York City, where I reveled in the pomp and ceremony of St. Patrick's Cathedral. The ritual of the mass calmed my brain and the warmth and light of the votive candles brought me closer to the higher power who could help me. Thank you to the people who paid for the many candles I lit each week.

In the winter of 1980 I finally made it to San Diego (my initial destination when I set out from St. Paul, Minnesota, that cold winter day in 1978). My newly repaired MG brought me to Mission Beach. At St. Brigid's Catholic Church in nearby Pacific Beach, Father Lloyd and

Father Richard welcomed me and introduced me to other young adults in a wonderful folk singing group. One of those members, Vanessa Puniak, remains a friend today. I remember that once Father Richard even dug unto his pockets for a $100 bill to pay for my car insurance. There, too, I met Beth Le Friant, who allowed me to camp out on her living room floor for a while. Then Northminster Presbyterian briefly became my church home; Bobbie McKee is still a friend today from that connection.

After I moved north to Encinitas, I was led to Christ Presbyterian Church of Rancho La Costa where I was first warmly welcomed by Interim Pastor Steve Jenks and Associate Pastor Ed Reynolds, PhD, and then later by Pastor Doug Kelly. I loved singing in the choir under the loving and forgiving leadership of Bergitta Brice and teaching Sunday school. It was so much fun to teach kids again! I still fondly remember Courtney and April Allen; the Artz girls: Erin, Kylie, and Aubrey; Laura and Megan Jones; Teddy Minner; and Allison and Martha Wright, who all ably assisted my teaching and didn't mind my non-adult behavior. There I was blessed with loving kindnesses especially by Dixie Jacobson and the Banes, Billings, Hayens, McCarters, Petersons, Wings; and dear, sweet MaryAnn Christ, who befriended me through all sorts of trials, took me to dinner, briefly housed me, walked with me on the beach, and listened and loved me. Another member, computer genius Reese Brown, volunteered to format and print the very first edition of *Brain Injury Rewiring* — all 86-pages! Thank you and bless you all!

Then the Episcopal Church — and more healing music — called me, first to St. Andrew's in Encinitas, then to St. Michael's in Carlsbad, and finally to St. Paul's Episcopal in Ventura and my beloved and supportive priest, Father Jerry Kahler. There was a brief interim stop at First Presbyterian in Santa Barbara, when I lived in my office (thank you to the lessee who kindly allowed me to sublet and sleep on the floor, while ignoring security reports!). Speaking of sleeping, without the Ventura Housing Authority and the Section 8 Program, I'd be homeless.

For brain rewiring, I first turned to school, starting with a study skills class and a reading improvement class way back in 1976. Building on my strengths is what the most notable professors did in my many ventures into the academic world. When my confidence allowed it, I began another graduate school program in counseling in the fall of 1977 at nearby University of Wisconsin at River Falls (UWRF). There I interacted with more wonderful, loving people.

One of my first post-injury professors, Dr. Vanetta Ogland, taught a psychology class entitled "Exceptional Children." After our first test, when I reported that I had over-studied, she responded, "All good students do." This was the very first time since the accident that I recall anyone ever telling me that I was good at anything. So I worked my tail off, loved her class, and even earned an A! She was the first one to call my writing "haunting," after she read one of my pieces about "The Boy from Avreyon," the story of the boy who lived in the wild and then was "saved" by some townspeople. (She noted my line "and he never smiled again.").

Also significant at UWRF was Bill Romoser, PhD, statistics professor, whose love for aphorisms kept me going ("It's tough to fly with eagles when you work for turkeys," and "Don't let the bastards get you down." (He said this in Latin to be PC, but I don't remember it.) Another was Counselor John Hamann, PhD, who took on the challenge of working with my psyche. John used my intellect and stubbornness to advantage, challenging me to overcome the demons. Without enough weapons, I couldn't yet, but his assistant, Joann introduced me to the desensitization techniques that would be very useful in many areas throughout my journey.

There were also special professors at Cal State Dominguez Hills, where I earned my first MA in Special Education in 1986. My adviser, Karl Skindrud, PhD, kindly helped me finish the program in ten months, while teaching full-time, even though when I told him my plan at our initial meeting, he said, "No one has ever done that." (I probably said, "Watch me," or something equally diplomatic.) Intellectual stimulation and emotional support in that program was provided by Judith Jackson, PhD, the language professor who actually made studying speech interesting.

After returning to San Diego and briefly teaching, I studied at San Diego State University from 1988-91. Special professors in the Physical Education Department (now known as Exercise Science) included Pete Aufsesser, PhD; Peggy Lasko-McCarthy, PhD; Tom McKenzie, PhD; and department chair, Rob Carlson, PhD. Another Midwest refugee, Pat

Patterson, PhD, who played the role of active guardian angel during my coursework, thesis work, and extensions, voluntarily chaired my thesis committee and worked with me weekly for nine months to restore my writing skills, develop a researcher's questioning mind, and befriend me generally. Uncannily, Pat could act knowledgeably, yet defer to me as the brain injury expert and allow me to develop the topic.

During my thirty-plus-year journey, I could always rely on physical activity to produce joy. And, while I've lifted weights in many different gyms across the country, my favorite indoor "fitness home" is the Ventura Family YMCA. The excitement that results from a wide diversity of ages is so refreshing. Not only am I thankful for the scholarship that allows me to be a member, but also for the accepting and happy feeling that permeates the facility. I don't mind that I'm often the only female in the free weight room either! Yoga Jones is my other indoor haven from stress.

Finally, I am very grateful to my brilliant and accommodating friends who supported my efforts and edited one or many chapters, starting again with Marlys Henke. Thank you, too, to my talented photographer, Don Anderson (with three PhDs!) and his able assistants, Joan Anderson and Susan Abrams, who are members of St. Paul's in Ventura. Actually, my entire church family, especially Kay Armstrong and the Leahys, deserve a huge thank you for supporting *Brain Injury Rewiring* and me for the past nine years! Many editors are church friends, including: Ralph Armstrong, MD, Bill Knutson, Dev Leahy (DevL), Larry Meyers, MD, and Jennie Whaley. Valuable help in dissecting dozens of research studies was provided by Diane Rennell, PhD, whom I met while ushering in Ventura. Thanks also to Mark Ylvisaker, PhD, who communicated with me for years despite battling melanoma; Rob Rich, DC, and John Dupler, PhD, for their chapter contributions; and early editors, Christine Baser, PhD, and Dan Gardner, MD, who labored over long chapters. For igniting the *Brain Injury Rewiring* spark, I'm indebted to the San Diego Brain Injury Foundation (SDBIF) for funding my initial thesis research and its former president Ron Ruff, PhD, for supporting it. Lastly, *Brain Injury Rewiring* would not even exist as a "New Connection" if not for the courage of Tom Blaschko of Idyll Arbor who persevered with me for five years from contract to final product. No doubt there were a few (or many) times he wondered about his own sanity during this adventure!

Throughout this thirty-plus-year journey, many other angels entered my life and offered their hearts, minds, backs, and, a few, even their pocketbooks, to lessen my load and lift me to the ledges beyond my reach. *Brain Injury Rewiring* is my thanks to you generous souls for your small and large acts of kindness. Know that others will reach the top because you first helped me. Bless you one and all!

Introduction

Life is a one-way street. No matter how many detours you take, none of them leads back. And once you know and accept that, life becomes much simpler. Because then you know you must do the best you can with what you have and what you are and what you have become.

— Isabel Moore

This *Brain Injury Rewiring for Loved Ones: A Lifeline to New Connections* is my gift of a helping hand to you as you join the work party in your survivor's challenge of a lifetime — his climb up the rehabilitation mountain.

In this *Lifeline*, you will learn the why, what and how of *rewiring* the brain and optimizing all systems — from the perspective of a long-term survivor. You will understand what to do and what to say — and not say — to him. You will read how to heal yourself and your family, too, as you all make new connections.

> Expect people to be better than they are; it helps them to become better. But don't be disappointed when they are not; it helps them to keep trying.
> — Merry Browne

I will show you how I grappled with — and overcame — the challenges by refusing to embrace the concept of *can't*. I'll show you how he can do this too, with your help! You will also see what research says about this most perplexing of injuries and the latest treatment methods to heal it.

This guidebook is half of a two-part set; your survivor will want his own *Lifeline* that empowers him to help himself and you. Transform your lives with the complete set: *Brain Injury Rewiring for Survivors* and *Brain Injury Rewiring for Loved Ones*!

1
Recollections of *the* Day

In the middle of the journey of our life, I came to myself in a dark wood where the straight path was lost.

— Dante

Old Highway 12, Inver Grove Heights, Minnesota
January 10, 1976, 11:37 AM

It happened on a snowy, blowy, winter day in Minnesota over three decades ago. As my mind flashed back to the ski lesson and ahead to seeing Hank, the friendly flurries of the morning gradually changed to gusts, and then to whiteout, obscuring the lane lines on Old Highway 12.

Soon the surface itself became almost invisible and I couldn't see if there even was a road! Every cell of my being focused on navigating my cherry-red MG Midget out of the turmoil of the storm and into the haven of my garage, just a few miles away.

Then, as snow blanketed the pavement and left me blizzard-blind, it happened — crash! My brain cannot remember and my soul cannot forget the collision. This is the conversation I had with myself that day:

"Boy, do I love to ski! It reminds me of cycling. Skis glide without effort, as I fly down hills, wind in my face, free — free to be. Actually, it's just great to be outside, exercising. I feel so alive, whole, happy — just being outdoors.

It's so unlike working at the hobby shop. What a bore! Hmmm, maybe I should call personnel on Monday and try teaching again; it sure wouldn't be boring. I'm just on extended sick leave, anyway.

3

Boy! Do I ever miss my old teaching job! I probably wouldn't have ulcers if I were still there. Darn it! What a great staff! We all really cared about one another, unlike that last place. What a switch! Still, despite no adult friends there, I liked most of the kids and even though the teaching wasn't as fun, the coaching, as always, was worth it. And working with the kids usually took my mind off the divorce.

God! I never thought divorce would be so awful, so lonely, so sad. But I just didn't like where our marriage was going and he refused to go to therapy with me. I suppose he thought he'd be outnumbered, me in a graduate program in counseling and all. I'm so sorry he didn't want to save it, not to mention shocked. I'll really miss his mother. God, I love her. I hope we can still be friends.

Well, my mother was right about John. I hate it when she's right! Sure am glad to have Hank in my life, but when is he going to be free? I guess I should be happy just to share what time we have. Can't wait to see him! All I have to do is watch for my exit. I'm almost there.

Okay, you're close. All you have to do is stay on the road. Find the exit. Are you in the right lane? Oops, better be sure. Go slowly, stay on the road."

That's all I remember. Now I am a survivor: someone who lived through an accident that caused a brain injury.

The Pre-Injury Person: Similarities Survivors Share

Many survivors and family members will recognize my chaotic life was similar to their own experiences. Although many of us would prefer to "idealize the deceased" — a psychological term for describing the pre-injury person as nearly perfect — research suggests that many survivors' lives immediately before the injury were lives of turbulence, disorder, and overwhelming risk-taking behavior.

That survivors share many similarities is well known: Those under age 30 incur 70% of all injuries, with males two to three times more likely to be involved than females. Survivors are four times more likely to be divorced and are unemployed more often than not. Significantly, nearly 75% of us survived a transport-related accident. Finally, the most significant contributing factor to all accidents is the use of alcohol, although not in my case — it was still morning!

On the spiritual side, if we survivors are honest about our pre-injury lives, there was no apparent life or focus of energy for many of us. The story you are about to read may not fit all survivors. It simply illustrates one kind of chaos — yours may have been different. We all came from different places, worked at different jobs, and may or may not have been in a loving relationship. But one thing we all share: we are now brain-injured, and our lives will never again be the same.

Revealing some of this history may tarnish my girl-next-door image for both old and new friends, but it's the truth — as far as I can remember. Facing that truth is vital for survivors to move past what was, to focus on what is, and what can be.

My Muddled Career and Emotional Life

Pre-injury, my life was a mess! Career, emotional, physical, and spiritual aspects were all in disarray, marked by questionable decisions that were likely influenced by alcohol and mostly prescription drugs — and maybe just a little "herb."

The structure that arises from a stable home and job life began to unravel, starting with a minor accident that resulted in a whiplash injury, for which I received cortisone injections and Valium prescriptions.

Then came the separation from my "until death do us part" husband of five years — a defining crack in my '50s and '60s fairy tale world that advertised: "Get a degree and follow that with an optional career. But be sure to marry, and make a home, and then live happily every after." Couples were supposed to agree on everything, and the fairy tale never told us what to do if incompatibility developed as people grew. After all, did Ozzie and Harriet ever fight?

In addition to the injury and the flaw in the marriage fairy tale, the fatal flaw ultimately proved to be in my workaday fairy tale: my teaching career at a beloved school was over. Reduced enrollment at the junior high where I taught, coached, counseled, and chaired the social committee forced an involuntary transfer.

In two months I lost both the security of a relatively stable home life and a very fulfilling work environment where I was loved, valued, and allowed to grow. This was followed by a bewildering summer filled with long walks and talks with friends that focused on the shock of a failed marriage. Graduate school, poetry workshops, and new friends from those endeavors helped ease the pain, but the summer's culminating move to a tiny apartment seemed to symbolize all that I lost. My new place lacked personality, pool, tennis courts — and my marriage partner. It visibly represented the emptiness that I felt.

The flaw in the fairy tale widened that fall and grew to a chasm when I realized that none of the features of my former beloved school — young, strong, close staff; programs that worked; energy; community support — were present in the new school. Perhaps more importantly, I was not a vital part of it. There was no reason to esteem newcomer me or seek my input. Still reeling from — and barely surviving — the losses, I was unable to find my role in this entrenched system, dashing my hope of a fresh career start.

At this school I met Hank, who pretended to be single, but wasn't, which I learned after I fell in love with him. The typical empty promise to get a divorce "...as soon as..." further disrupted the fairy tale.

Hospitalization for an ulcer attack interrupted this confusing scene, first on a medical floor — then on the psychiatric wing! After a bewildering month, I was released and found a special position at an experimental school offering strong people and energy, but not the structure and belonging I so desperately needed.

After vagabonding between the homes of parents and various friends, I moved back to the same apartment building of my married life, and began the next year at yet another school I didn't like, which had even fewer of the qualities I valued.

Then another hospitalization. This time it was straight to the psychiatric ward — for depression and ulcers again. As part of my treatment plan, doctors recommended I take an extended sick leave from my now very unfulfilling teaching career and work part-time in sales at a nearby hobby shop. This sounded appropriate for two reasons: I was born to sell and the sales job would be less stressful. But it lacked vitality, even at Christmas, and I missed teaching, missed the kids — and missed the feeling of doing something worthwhile.

During this tumultuous year and a half, my support network — parents, family, friends — were still dealing with the fact I was no longer part of a couple — my parents reacted with anger and my friends and family with avoidance. After they initially comforted me, I lost my close circle of loved ones. Most old friends were temporarily out of touch at this time — everyone struggled with their own issues.

My only spiritual life was that found at the end of a bong or in a bottle of Scotch, in bed, or behind the wheel of my cherished red MG Midget. I vaguely remember a bit — maybe a lot — of sexual acting-out. Physically, I was not able to consistently exercise. Still suffering with whiplash from two minor accidents — before the MG — I took Valium at will and often washed it down with an alcoholic beverage while out socializing. Besides this self-medication, I randomly took other drugs that doctors prescribed for depression. Did I mention a certain fondness for marijuana in a wine-filled bong?

The pre-injury portrait you've just read paints a life in turmoil, to be sure. Career and marriage lost, our girl-next-door was struggling — and losing. Although my memory is somewhat cloudy, it's likely that I simply do not recall other disturbing events, probably in an unconscious attempt to maintain some semblance of dignity — I ask your understanding for that. But even with no other contributing factors, you get the picture. It is not surprising that I was an accident waiting to happen. I do vividly remember the following scene at the hospital — terror does that.

After the Injury, Ramsey Medical Center St. Paul, Minnesota January 10, 1976, 6:11 PM

Where am I? Why is everything dark? Hank and I were supposed to meet at noon. What are my parents doing here, standing over by that window? My mother looks worried. She's wearing that frown and my father looks distressed — I guess. I've never seen that look on his face before. It's sort of mad and sad at the same time.

Oh, God! What's the matter with me? Why can't I move? Why am I strapped down? Why does my head hurt? Why does everything hurt? Why can't I talk? Am I dead? Where am I? Why am I in this gown, in this bed, in this strange, dark room? Why are my parents looking at me like that?

I want to say, "Hi!" and smile, so my mother will stop frowning — but I can't, so I moan. They look at me and Mom says, "Honey, you're in the hospital and you had a bad car accident, but the doctor says you'll be fine."

Oh God, No! Not my MG — my precious MG — not my MG!

That's all I remember. That — and the absolute terror of not being able to speak.

End of Day 1

Beginning of the climb — the endless climb — the climb that demands your all — the climb that either kills you or makes you strong.

2
Climbing the Mountain

This time it's make or break. All senses concentrate. He knows that's what it takes. For a victory. Only the strongest survive. No room for compromise. He races with the time. And his own mortality. Some people don't know how to give in. You knock 'em down. They just pick themselves up again. And all they got is. Willpower. To make a dream come true. Don't underestimate willpower. It can move a mountain or two...

— G. Lyle, T. Britten

The crash forever changed my concentration — from navigating my beloved MG to navigating myself through the windy, tortuous switchbacks that meander up the mountain of life. I describe my more than 30-year ascent in the following story, where an avalanche substitutes for the car crash.

Today, my climb up the mountain continues, on the surface not all that different from others navigating through the ordinary switchbacks of their lives. But after an avalanche interrupted my previous expedition, careening me onto a rocky ledge, several things do distinguish me from my fellow travelers. Now my brain needs direct commands and half of my body wants to rest while the other half works. And although I look fine, neither my repaired equipment nor my old clothes seem to fit. Funny how no one else notices.

Other members of my hiking party move faster than I. They question my slow pace; I look like I'm in shape for this journey, except for a few cuts and bruises.

It's at times like these that I wish for a defining scar of some sort, a visible sign of my limits, like a big "HI" for "head-injured" prominently displayed on my forehead. Then maybe people would give me a break. And I could give myself a break. But they'd probably see it as a greeting and say, "Hi!" — or ask for an explanation that could lead me to an outburst, which would just make everything worse. As it is, I look fine.

No one gives me credit for surviving the near-fatal avalanche, rehabilitating myself, and setting out on yet another climb. What does happen, however, is that other hikers frequently nag me to move faster and tell me to lighten my load if I can't make it. They offer suggestions that begin with "Why don't you just …" and say, "You don't look disabled to me." Funny how no one asks me if I have a problem.

Exasperated at my halting steps, one of the leaders places an extra sun visor on my head, convinced that the bright sun is slowing my progress. But the hat slips down my sweaty forehead, covers my good eye, and I'd have to drop the lifeline to fix it. Now the only visible direction is down, the crooked hat masks my tears, and I struggle even more. Funny how no one sees this.

Some fellow climbers doubt my efforts and challenge my courage. "What's the matter, why can't you keep up? My pack is bigger than yours. You said you were a tough athlete." This is followed by more "Why don't you just …" suggestions with variations on the "Try a little harder!" theme. Oh, I wish I had that scar and didn't look so fine. But still, it's funny how no one tries to understand.

The other hikers offer many suggestions except for the one that would help — offering to carry part of my load. Perhaps because each pack has been custom-designed, no one wants to take part of my pack's weight, create an imbalance, and jeopardize his own success. Funny about that.

Everyone tells me how much easier it would be if I had been able to save my original equipment. No kidding. This is followed by marveling at how lucky I was to survive with so little damage and how good I look. Sporting a very large scar increases in appeal by the minute. Then maybe they'd commend me for my efforts — perhaps even ask how to help me.

As it is, as they continue their climbs, they laugh at the repaired gear that hasn't adjusted to my new shape. I force a smile to avoid the extra burden of an outburst, try to hold back my tears, and talk to God and to myself.

"Remember, 'Act as if' — as if you're not weak, not inadequate, as if you can do it." I stumble on, but without laughing. It's not funny.

Maybe they forget that I, too, loved my original form-fitting pack. I need to remember that they mean well, and that at least we're still on the journey together. After all, they haven't asked me to leave their group — yet. I hope they remember that I'm doing the best I can. Funny how no one offers to change places with me. And I don't even have a scar. *"It could be worse. I could be falling or stuck at the bottom or alone."*

Suddenly, there's a shelf and a hand reaches down to help pull me up. The sun and the other hikers warmly greet me. My tears are over, for now, replaced by a smile and a thank-you. The next ledge is in view and the mountaintop — shrouded by clouds since the beginning of the climb — actually looks reachable. Funny about that.

My Three Helping Hands

Most survivors likely will empathize with this story — and also understand that everyone carries a loaded backpack. Hopefully, most loved ones and professionals will help to carry part of our load. Indeed, what we all really need to climb the mountain is a helping hand.

To explain why I now mostly peer down at the vista below me instead of being mired in the muck at the bottom or marooned on an obscure ledge on the mountainside, I can think of three reasons:

- God, church, and my religious family — my spiritual life.
- Willpower, hard work, and achievable goals — my values, beliefs, and attitudes.
- Friends and family — my support system.

All of these are interdependent, e.g., many friends are from my religious family — and none of them could carry the extra load alone.

Even with God on my side, if there were no God's helpers or no Minnesota work ethic, my journey would likely have ended long ago. For any significant, lasting progress to occur I still need them all.

A good example of all my helpers working together followed my running a 5K race, attended by members of my adopted San Diego family. A 20-foot high rock-climbing wall attracted the teenager in our family. Because there would be over an hour's wait, I agreed to stand in the long line with him. As we stood there, I noticed that most of the other climbers were between 10 and 40 years younger than I. Two women only a decade or so younger cajoled me into climbing, too. They even requested that I climb first since I had run the race and looked to be in shape.

My anxiety increased as we neared the wall. Questions peppered my mind: *"Where are they placing their limbs to successfully climb? What doesn't work? How did that kid race up the wall so fast? Why doesn't anyone here look remotely close to my age? Why am I so anxious — don't I always say I love to try new things — am I becoming conservative? What would be the worst thing that could happen?"*

The teenager was next and quickly scampered to the top. It was my turn. *"OK, use the holds that the others did. Good! Hands and feet are in place. Oops, now what?"* After one more move, my face nearly touched the wall, every muscle in my body was tense, I was stretched to the limit — and I was stuck.

Seeing the panicked look on my face, family members loudly cheered. As this power surged through me, I scanned the wall for places to move to. Then — luckily — the staff person advised me where to place my left foot. *"Way over there?"* I said to myself. It seemed too far to stretch, but I didn't have another alternative, so attempted the reach — and happily found myself stretching farther than I ever imagined I could!

The rest of the climb was easy, and I reached the top to ring the bell and cheer loudly. *"Wow! After that one obstacle, it was easy to succeed!"* Thanks to all the helpers, I made it — my first wall-climbing experience was a success!

This rock-climbing wall is a metaphor for survivors climbing the recovery mountain: if we stretch farther than we think we can, we can achieve; if we prepare, we can succeed; if at first we don't succeed, try,

try again. Sometimes we may need to just have faith that help is there, even if we cannot see it. The obstacle needn't defeat us just because it looks impassable. We need all of our helpers to work at the same time in order to succeed.

My teenage friend and I moved on to the more advanced wall with confidence. There we were able to place our hands in holds that we could not see after the helpers assured us those were the ones we

> The distance doesn't matter; only the first step is difficult.
> — Mme. du Deffand

needed. We believed them because they had been correct earlier and there appeared to be no other holds that would work anyway. In fact, all the crevices seemed to shrink as we reached them! Thanks to all working together, we climbed up this wall faster than the first and easier one, clanged the bell, and cheered.

Can survivors use my experience on their mountain climbs? Will others see my success and gain enough courage to either start their climbs or continue their journeys with more resolve and confidence? That's my hope.

December 1978 — and the rest of my life

I'll never forget my prognosis after I was injured in 1976: "suicide or psych ward." I remember being both surprised and shocked by what they said. Here I was, a schoolteacher, someone who believed in the power of education to change lives, and they wrote me off! Not only did I wonder what those %?$*&#! were on, but it motivated me to prove them wrong! And it still does — this is why I am writing this book!

Just because I seemed to favor both the excitement of driving an MG and occasionally the security of the psychiatric hospital didn't necessarily make me suicidal and schizophrenic! I simply needed to find my purpose and focus again — to start over — following a period of living on the edge, walking with the devil, and feeling adrift.

After my world blew up, I needed to replace it — with something better! My two years of trauma — including failed suicide attempts — only reaffirmed my belief that, as my childhood friend Louise said,

"You're here for a reason, Carolyn." My mission was to find that purpose before my capabilities were lessened any more.

To prepare for any mission, an inventory needs to be taken: What do I have? What do I need? Where am I going? What do I seek?

Before I could "go with God," I needed to see my way through a dilemma: if God doesn't make junk, why do I feel like it? A typical God response — unpredictable and provocative — arrived at a freeway exit stoplight:

"Child, you were chosen, not discarded. And I chose you because you are strong. Many others are not as strong as you, so you need to help them to carry their load — and I will help you to carry yours. Remember, Jesus already took the big rap. You don't need to carry all of it, too. I'm not asking you to do that. What I am asking is for you to be the best you that you can be. And, when you feel down, remember how tough you are. It is because you are tough that I ask a bit more of you. I will not ask you to do more than you are able. Just call on me when you feel weak and, together, we will prevail. Just remember to call on me."

I paused. My thinking did a 180° turn — from feeling discarded to feeling chosen. So, that's why all the hell — to prove to myself how strong I was. Then, my first positive self-talk in a long time: "You must be pretty damn tough to withstand all that you have faced. And, you have prevailed!"

After this awakening, I could proceed to answer my mission questions: What do we have? What do we need? Where are we going? Why? What if?

First, what I had: cold Minnesota, with snow, ice, scary roads, and six weeks — maybe — of summer complete with the "State Bird" — the mosquito; Mom and Dad — but they're gone all the time, especially in the winter; Aunt Chelsie, Marlys, Louise, and Mary Ellen; bad memories of accident, rape, and school lay-off; vocational/academic failure, and the cabin.

Second, what I needed: something better. With warm weather, ocean, and freedom from snow and cold and scary roads. A fresh start. A graduate school for social work.

Third, where am I going? Either California or Hawaii is warm and provides both the ocean and appropriate graduate schools.

Fourth, why? What if? I can and I must. It is suicide to stay. I need to be free of the snow, the bad memories. If I don't like it, I can always return. Go now before the worst of the snow and cold. This is reminder enough that I must go or I'll die here, unfulfilled.

So, one cold, snowy, winter day in December of 1978, I left Minnesota. One warm, sunny, winter day in December of 1980, I arrived in the Mission Beach community of San Diego, California. A snowdrift in southern Minnesota waylaid me, and the same Rocky Mountain blizzards that blocked the shortest route led me to my wonderful El Paso shrink DJ. It was a two-year journey — a lifetime of experiences that can be revisited at will.

It wasn't easy or fast. But it did happen and it's still happening. I remember my first race of any kind in twenty years: I cycled thirty miles in just over an hour and a half (1:34) to place second to an All-American triathlete in my over-50 age group in a bicycle road race! My new built-up cycling shoes with special inserts actually provided me with two good legs. The result was a shock — no pain and no flats — and I had not trained! Imagine what will happen when I do! When's the next race?!

My recovery over these past thirty-plus years has, in some ways, been nothing short of a miracle — if the many brushes with death and further injury encountered on this journey are considered. In writing this book, even I am amazed at the outcome after all my adventures!

My Invitation to You

Come with me now as we all climb this mountain together. Let's explore how to help mend our survivor's equipment and even help him make his peace with it from time to time. Let's help treat his wounds

> Don't underestimate willpower. It can move a mountain or two.
> — G. Lyle, T. Britten

and reduce his stumbles. Let's help him reach the top — or at least higher than anyone thought he could. Let's also lighten the loads of our fellow travelers — we know what a difference that can make. Eventually, when he begins to hike more and stumble less, and after he reaches a ledge or two, we'll all breathe easier. Maybe all of us will even enjoy the rest of the climb!

3
Brain Construction and Wiring

It is the wounded oyster that mends its shell with pearl.

— Ralph Waldo Emerson

After your survivor's injury, you probably ask questions like these: "How are our brains constructed and wired?" "What happens when a healthy brain is damaged?" "How are injuries diagnosed and treated?" "What behaviors usually result?" "How do brains recover?" "What does my loved one need to do to rewire?" "How can we help?"

Keep asking! This chapter summarizes what experts tell us about the brain and its wiring, the effects of brain injury, and recovery and rewiring in general:

Brain 101: Structure and wiring. Basic information about brain structure, function, and wiring of the communication system.

Brain 102: Injuries, damage, and effects. Information about the different kinds of injuries and sites.

Brain 103: Treatments and tests. Various diagnostic instruments and procedures that might be used in his evaluation and care.

Brain 104: General recovery/rewiring questions — if, when, how, and why. How the brain recovers, what behaviors you can expect, and what you can do to help.

Introduction

Brain injured or not, everything in our environment impacts us, either positively or negatively, to a greater or lesser degree. People, places, or things — prescription medications, street drugs, alcohol, food, exercise, or any physical, mental, emotional, or spiritual interaction — can either enhance or diminish us.

Your survivor's brain chemistry is especially sensitive. Help him be kind to himself. Help him to refrain from polluting himself internally and to avoid polluting himself externally with toxic people, places, and things. To help you understand the inner workings of the brain and how to help him, let's begin with the mental part — rewiring.

Brain 101: Structure and Wiring

What is the structure of the brain?

The three main sections of the brain are

- The *cerebrum*, "the seat of consciousness," the center for higher mental faculties, such as thinking and feeling, and all voluntary muscular activities.
- The *cerebellum*, located at the base of the skull, responsible for coordination of voluntary muscular movements.
- The *brain stem*, located deep in the brain, connects the left and right sides of the cerebrum with the spinal cord, responsible for basic functions of consciousness and life maintenance, such as breathing and heart rate.

What are the parts of the *cerebrum* and what activities do they control?

Divided into an outer layer called the *cerebral cortex* and an inner layer called the *subcortex*, the *cerebrum* can also be divided into right and left sides called *cerebral hemispheres*.

The outer layer *cerebral cortex* as a whole controls our perceptions and actions, our spoken and written language, and our abilities to think, reason, plan, and act.

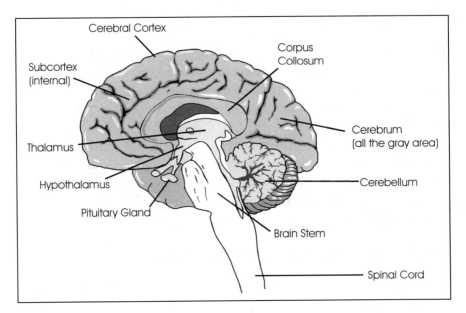

Figure 1: Internal structures of the brain.

The inner layer *subcortex* includes the *limbic system*, which regulates emotional experience and expression; the *thalamus*, which is an important sensory relay station; and the *hypothalamus*, which regulates such basic functions as sleep, sex drive, hunger, thirst, and emotional response. The *hypothalamus* also controls the *pituitary gland*, the body's master gland that regulates the endocrine hormone system.

Divided by a deep, lengthwise fissure, or crevice, the *cerebral hemispheres* command specific responsibilities. The *left hemisphere* controls the right side of the body and guides language processing plus analytic and verbal thinking. The *right hemisphere* directs the left side of the body and oversees spatial and whole-concept thinking plus creative and musical activities.

How are the *hemispheres* connected? How are their duties divided?
A thick layer of crosswise nerve fibers called the *corpus callosum* interconnects the hemispheres so that almost every part of one hemisphere links with the corresponding part of the other.

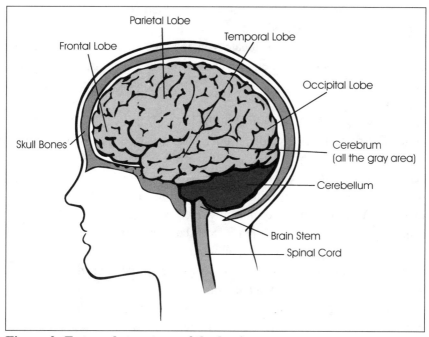

Figure 2: External structure of the brain.

Each hemisphere is divided into four sections called *lobes.* The largest is the *frontal lobe,* at about one-third of the total brain volume. The other lobes are the *parietal, temporal,* and *occipital.*

Located on the front part of the brain, right behind the forehead, the *frontal lobes* organize behavior. The functions controlled by the *frontal lobes* include emotional regulation and reaction, attention, judgment, and motor control. *Executive function* is a term often used to describe *frontal-lobe* abilities, describing the duties of our "brain-boss" which directs the complicated activities required by a thinking human being. This administrator is responsible for putting into effect complex, goal-directed activities — like preparing a meal — that require detailed planning to achieve a purpose.

The *parietal lobes* are located near the sides and top of the head. Their functions include interpretation of bodily sensations, visual/spatial perception, perception of position in space (*proprioception*) and numerical reasoning needed to do arithmetic.

The *temporal lobes* are located on the side of the head above the ears, by the temples. Their functions include hearing — auditory processing of sounds, language, and music, memory, and emotional expression.

The *occipital lobes* are found at the back of the head by the occipital bone. Their functions include visual scanning and processing, reading, and facial recognition. A large amount of the brain relative to the other senses is devoted to processing vision.

To summarize: the back portions are more involved with receiving input; the front portions are more involved with sending output, and the central portions are where input is translated into output. From outside in, the brain is organized from integrated, complex, general conscious activities in the *cortex*, to more automatic, reflexive, and individualized activities in the *subcortex* and *medulla*.

Even though the brain is divided into hemispheres and lobes, it functions as a whole and is more complex than an advanced computer! All of its component parts are wired to interact with one another continuously to produce our complex activities. Unlike a computer, the human brain is constantly changing. It does not need to be externally updated or replaced by a better version. The various programs don't need to be turned on separately — the human brain is always on!

What does the brain look like?

The brain is a soft mass of interconnecting tracts that looks like unset gray pudding (grey matter) surrounding white yogurt (white matter). The gray matter contains numerous neuronal cell bodies and synapses. The white matter is composed of many fiber pathways.

Together, the brain and spinal cord weigh about three pounds. The entire mass of the brain can fit in the palm of an average-sized adult's hand. Neither brain size nor head size indicate how "smart" the brain is. Only the depth and number of neuronal connections can determine intelligence!

What kinds of cells are located there in the brain?

The brain is composed of two principal types of brain cells, *neurons* and *glia.* An average brain starts out with about 100 billion *neurons,* which are the most complicated and among the largest cells in the body with some parts that may stretch as long as a yard.

Our *neurons* function to process and convey information, working together in both local and long-distance circuits. Some *neurons* receive information not just from other areas within the brain and spinal cord, but from many different parts of the body. In fact, a single *neuron* may connect with as many as 10 million other neurons throughout the brain (Stein, Brailowsky, & Will, 1995).

Neurons consist of three parts: a *soma* (cell body), *dendrites* (branchlike projections) that cover the *soma,* and *axons* (longer cable-like nerve fibers). The ends of the *axons* branch out to look like plant roots, except that the ends of the rootlets, called *axon terminals,* look like little feet and act like communication terminal buttons. These feet release and reabsorb the chemicals used by the *neurons* to communicate with one another. Each *neuron* may be linked to other neurons by thousands of *synapses* (connections between *axons* and *axon terminals).*

Glia (also called *glial cells*) are non-*neuron* brain cells that serve the vital function of co-directing *neurons* to their targets. Outnumbering *neurons* ten to one, *glial cells* also insulate and protect the *axon.* They can divide and reproduce themselves throughout life. They store nutrients that *neurons* use throughout life to grow and function. They help to repair damage to neurons. They manufacture and store *neurotransmitters* — the *neurons* use these chemicals to communicate with each other.

How is the brain protected physically?

Like a precious castle surrounded by a moat, the brain is well protected by several layers of membranes called *meninges.* The layers of the *meninges* — the *pia,* the *arachnoid,* and the *dura* — form a pad between the brain and the skull.

The *pia* is a thin and vascular layer that hugs the surface of the brain. The middle layer is the *arachnoid,* which acts like a spider web between the *meninges* and the *pia.* Directly lining the skull is the *dura,* which is a thick, inelastic, and durable double-layered membrane. Separating the two layers of the *dura* are thick venous channels called *sinuses*. The smooth inner layer of the *dura* sends four parts inward into the cavity of the skull to support and protect the different parts of the brain and forms sheaths for the nerves that pass through the openings in the skull. The rough outer layer of the *dura* adheres tightly to the inner surface of the skull bones.

The final layer of physical protection is the skull — a bony frame-work of eight cranial bones, 14 facial bones, and the teeth. Except for the lower jaw, the skull is immovable. *Sutures* (fibrous tissue) make uneven-appearing connections that meet like map pieces between the bones of the cranium and face. The inside of the skull looks like a mountain range with varying peaks and valleys covered with the moss of the *dura*.

In what other ways is the brain protected?

A multi-layered system helps to maintain the balance of the brain chemistry, starting with the *blood-brain barrier (BBB)*. This intricate network, a membrane of *glial cells* wrapped around blood vessels, is the first wall of defense between the body's circulating blood and the brain. It acts like a filtering system, preventing certain damaging substances from reaching brain tissue and the *cerebrospinal fluid (CSF)* — a watery liquid that cushions the brain and spinal cord from physical impact.

Surrounding all brain cells is a moist environment that contains a variety of chemicals and nutrients that originate in a variety of ways: made and released by the *neurons* themselves, released from other support cells, filtered from the blood supply, and from the *CSF*. After trauma, *CSF* may leak and usually changes from a clear fluid to one with a yellowish or reddish tint.

This complex chemical soup plays a role in controlling and modify-ing the flow of information from one cell to another throughout the body. As a result of these widely available chemicals, distant sites in the brain can be affected, even indirectly, by the activity of one *neuron*. For example, muscle tension can affect the taste of food.

Two main pairs of arteries supply the brain with nutrients and similar veins drain the used blood away from the brain. The carotid arteries run up each side inside the front of the neck, accompanied by the carotid veins. Similarly, the vertebral arteries and veins run along side one another inside each side of the back of the neck. Blood normally flows up all four arteries, equalizing pressure. *CSF* circulates throughout the skull and collects in the *dural sinuses*. Venous blood drains directly from the eye into the cavernous sinus. All the brain's veins drain into the internal jugular vein.

How is the intact (non-injured) brain wired?

Simply put, the brain is wired like a telephone system: a call from one party travels along the line (the *axon* of a *neuron*) through the chemical soup until its *axon terminal* connects with its chosen receiver *neuron(s)*. *Neurons* communicate with one another within the brain and throughout the body by interconnections called *synapses*. All of our internal and external communication flows through two kinds of *synapses*. These *synapses* form and reform continuously, billions of times every minute of our lives.

Two kinds of *synapses, electrical* and *chemical*, link the *neurons*. All signals begin their journey as electrical impulses that speed down the *axon*, carrying the message like a telephone cable. The *polarized* (unidirectional) impulse that travels down the first *neuron* starts an impulse in the second *neuron* and so on, like a chain reaction. The stronger the triggering event, the greater the frequency or rate of nerve impulses that travel down the *axon*. For example, a strong signal like hearing an explosion causes a higher number of nerve impulses than hearing a cat's meow.

Electrical synapses occur in some parts of the brain where neurons are tiny, dense, have short *axons* (cables) and few *dendrites* (projections), and where the signal passes directly from one cell to another without the chemical transformation that is typical of most *neurons*. These are mostly local calls. The activity of *electrical synapses* is like that of a symphony conductor directing and fine-tuning the impulses that travel down neighboring cells.

Chemical synapses are more numerous, more capable of adapting to environmental changes, more sensitive to foreign agents (for example, medications), and show a greater variety of responses than *electrical synapses*.

When an impulse arrives at a cell, *calcium ions* (one of the nutrients found outside the cell) rush through a tiny opening in the membrane of the *axon terminal.* This opening was created by the electrical impulse when it arrived. This flow of *calcium ions* into the terminals starts another chain reaction: *neurotransmitters* are released into the space between the two *neurons* and fuse to *receptor proteins,* special sites on the adjacent cell that are manufactured by the *neurons.* A *neurotransmitter's* receptor may also team with special molecules to form a second messenger system. In this case, the *neurotransmitter,* acting as the first messenger, hands off to an intracellular second messenger.

To simplify: a *neuron* hurls a ball (*neurotransmitter*) at the glove (*axon*) of a second neuron. The ball is caught only if the catcher is looking and the glove is at the right place (*synapse*) at the right time. If there is a communication breakdown, numerous other less desirable possibilities may occur: the ball could land in the dugout, carom off the umpire, or be caught by an outfielder or even a fan in the stands!

How do neurotransmitters work?

These gatekeepers help determine if the *neurons* are receptive to the impulse to *stimulate* (excite) the next neuron or *inhibit* (block) it, either transporting the impulse or not.

The *neurotransmitters* (for example, *serotonin, dopamine,* and *acetylcholine*) work like a key that fits into a lock (*receptor*). The *receptors* allow the *neurotransmitters* and other substances to alter the surrounding nerve membrane and permit the *ions* (sodium, potassium, calcium, and chloride) to flow freely in and out of the cell. In turn, when the *ions* flow into and out of the *neurons*, they set up electrical currents.

The more impulses that arrive, the more *neurotransmitters* flow out of the *axon terminals* and the easier it is to start an impulse in the next set of *neurons.* As *neurotransmitters* are released and attach to the membrane, the local current increases until an impulse is generated that either stimulates or inhibits a neighboring *neuron's* activity.

If the impulse is stimulated, it then rushes down the nerve's *axon* to produce changes in the *axon terminals.* This process is continuously repeated throughout life. *Neurons* dynamically modify their synaptic connections in response to genetic programming, chemicals, diseases, and all of life's experiences — which is how we learn!

Sometimes it's better if nerve impulses do not get through. Some *neurotransmitters* slow down or stop the transmission of signals. Like the ebb and flow of the ocean, the interaction between exciting and inhibiting a nerve modulates the flow of impulses in the *neuron*. It is normal for nerve cell activity to be inhibited; in some cases, it is necessary. For example, certain interfering noises, like background noise in a restaurant, need to be blocked in order to listen to someone talking. Many survivors experience problems screening out stimuli. They react, or overreact, to almost everything. Some find that they function better when they take medication like Prozac or Zoloft — known as *selective serotonin reuptake inhibitors (SSRIs)*. For these survivors, the *SSRI* may do the job their brains cannot do on their own — block out noise.

Brain 102: Injuries, Damage, and Effects

Let's review what we know about the healthy brain: *neurons* communicate like a telephone system where each cable is protected to maintain the strength and integrity of the system. The *blood-brain barrier (BBB)* is our first wall of defense. The layers of the *BBB* act as filters and help to maintain balance.

What happens when a healthy brain is injured?

A chain reaction or cascade of events occurs that alters the balance of the brain chemistry. Even if the area that is damaged is small, the entire brain is affected if the *BBB* has been invaded or broken down. When the *BBB* is violated, a flood of blood cells, proteins, and other substances fill the cellular spaces usually reserved for *neurons* and *glia*. Just like any other unexpected and unwanted flood, the fluid builds rapidly and the brain swells. This swelling is called *edema*. The *glial cells* act like sponges to protect the *neurons* from the flood of toxins caused by the injury, but they swell, too. They absorb fluids — they cannot stop the flow of the flood. When the *glial* cells get overloaded, they die, and then toxic substances are re-released into the circulation, thereby killing more *glia* and *neurons*. Chaos reigns. Every living cell reacts with shock. The brain tries to fight back and to adjust to the invasion.

In spite of the trauma, the injured cells do everything in their power to live. *Neurotransmitters* and their activating agent, *calcium ions*, are released. This now-toxic spill kills vulnerable neurons by overexciting them or damaging them because their membranes are overloaded. Highly electrically charged particles (*free radicals*) can now freely roam and attack brain cell membranes at will — brain stability is imperiled. The longer the flood continues, the more damage and functional impairment result. What was a balanced, nourishing soup is now a dangerously toxic soup. Where healthy cells once received proper nourishment and oxygen from intact blood vessels, the ruptured blood vessels can no longer transport the elements critical to the survival of all the brain cells. More cell death occurs.

How does the injury affect the communication system?
Electrical impulses sent from *neuron* to *neuron* are interrupted and signals are incomplete. Portions of the brain may no longer communicate with one another, either totally or partially, or signals may move at a much slower speed. Disruptions can involve both processing speed and ability. In the case of a severe injury, some neurons actually die; other neurons may be active, but no longer as efficient.

What are the different kinds of acquired brain injuries and damage?
Common types of injury are *traumatic brain injury* (TBI) and *cerebrovascular accident* (CVA), also called *stroke*. (A less common problem that also causes injury to healthy brain cells is *brain tumor.*) The type and site of injury and how the injury occurred determine the kind and amount of damage that is sustained and whether that damage is *focal* or *diffuse*. Damage may be caused by increased pressure on brain tissue and/or physical disruption of the brain.

Focal damage is local to a particular area of the brain and usually produces specific patterns of deficits that correspond to the functions controlled by the damaged tissue. For example, it is common for a right-hemisphere stroke or other injury to produce inattention/neglect on the left side of the body because the right side of the brain controls the left side of the body. Both internal traumatic events, e.g., from *stroke* or *brain tumor* and external events, such as a gunshot wound or skull fracture, may produce *focal damage.*

Diffuse damage to the brain may be widespread or scattered and is caused by rotational forces resulting from abrupt acceleration and deceleration as the head turns on top of the flexible neck. The *axons* (the parts of the *neurons* that connect the different areas of the brain) are vulnerable to injury during high-speed accidents when there is twisting and turning of the brain around the brain stem, The physical forces that are produced stretch and shear (tear apart) each *axon* in the affected area..

What happens during a traumatic brain injury (TBI)?
Major chaos erupts, as in natural disasters such as earthquakes that can involve many people, except in this case the many people are *neurons.* Some *neurons* die instantly, some are mortally wounded and die soon, others suffer serious injuries yet stay alive, and still others — the lucky ones — escape all harm. Some of the surviving cells look normal, appear unscathed, but are actually weakened and susceptible to stress overload — and the dysfunction that accompanies it — throughout their lives.

There are two kinds of TBI: *head injuries* can be *open* and *closed,* referring to the injury's effect on the skull rather than on the brain. Both kinds can cause concussions that result in similar trauma to the brain. A closed head injury may result in a depressed skull fracture — a dent in the skull — in which the broken bone presses into the brain.

How do *open-head injuries* differ from *closed-head injuries*?
In an *open-head injury* the skull is penetrated, exposing the brain and leaking brain tissue to the outside of the head. Typical examples include gunshot, shrapnel, or stab wounds. Penetration of the skull forces hair, skin, and bone fragments into the brain, increasing the risk of infection. Gunshot wounds cause further primarily focal damage as bullets ricochet within the skull, causing shock waves inside the brain and widening the area of destruction. This usually produces specific patterns of deficits that correspond to the functions controlled by the damaged tissue in a particular brain lobe or area.

In a *closed-head injury,* no penetration of the skull occurs. The force of the trauma transfers directly to the brain within the closed, bony surfaces inside the skull. This may result in more *diffuse damage* than in an *open-head injury* and may or may not be more severe than *focal* damage. Typical examples include hitting the dashboard/windshield or being struck with a blunt weapon, like football helmets colliding or taking a punch from a boxer's fist. The results are often described as *coup-countercoup* (blow-counterblow) injuries.

A *coup* injury occurs at the impact site when the head suddenly stops and the brain is propelled forward against the skull, rubbing and bumping against the inner ridges. A *countercoup* injury results from rebound trauma: after the brain bounces off the original impact site, it bumps against the opposite side of the skull and rubs along the inner bony projections. Another description of this wound is an acceleration-deceleration injury.

Closed-head injuries are often referred to as *concussions,* which is a temporary loss or lessening of consciousness caused by either a direct blow on the head or an indirect injury due to rotational forces. In both mild and more severe *concussions* microscopic nerve and blood vessel harm may occur although there may be no damage visible to the naked eye or on neuroimaging tests like the MRI.

How are the different kinds of closed head injuries rated?
Severity is rated using neurological criteria such as the Glasgow Coma Scale (GCS) and by documenting loss of consciousness (LOC) and *post-traumatic amnesia* (loss of memory after the injury). Brain damage is classified from very mild to very severe. Typically, mild injuries score 13-15 on the GCS with LOC for less than 60 minutes; moderate head injuries score nine to twelve on the GCS with LOC of from one to 24 hours; and severe injuries score less than eight on the GCS with more than 24 hours of LOC. In general, the more severe the head injury, the more profound the brain damage and resulting disability. However, many additional factors, such as pre-injury personality and physical status, influence outcome.

What types of damage occurs in the most common sites of injury?
Closed-head injuries typically injure the *frontal* and the *temporal lobes*, due to the size of the *frontal* lobes and closeness of both lobes to the inwardly projecting bony portions of the skull that they rub against during trauma. Additionally, the physical forces of the trauma throughout the brain can cause *axonal injury* (stretching or shearing along the neuron) which affects neurotransmitter systems, producing resultant deficit areas that are as varied as the physical, cognitive, and psychosocial functions that the brain itself supports.

Closed-head trauma causes two types of damage. *Primary damage* is caused at the time of trauma from physical forces applied to the brain. *Secondary damage* develops from complications from the primary trauma. Perhaps the most serious and complex injuries result from *inner cerebral trauma* due to *diffuse axonal injury* (DAI) caused by coup-countercoup injuries. This common damage necessitates rewiring because brain messages are lost or slowed after *axons* are damaged. Additionally, *contusions* (bruising) and *hematomas* (blood clots) are likely to occur, causing further damage.

Secondary damage may occur anywhere from seconds to days after the actual impact. Damaged blood vessels may block blood flow leading to *hypoxia/anoxia* (lack of oxygen in the brain), or they may rupture and cause a *hemorrhage* (bleeding) which can lead to a *hematoma* that forms within the cranial cavity. Blood and fluids from ruptured vessels cause *edema* (swelling) and increase *intracranial pressure.*

To understand *intracranial pressure*, imagine a rigid suitcase or box that is stuffed too full: the contents spill out or create bulges. The added pressure from swollen brain tissue, blood, and *cerebrospinal fluid* overfills the rigid bony skull. Because the skull can't stretch like skin, the increasing pressure compresses the skull contents.

Increased intracranial pressure on the brain stem can lead to *seizures,* unconsciousness, cardiorespiratory distress, or brain herniation (where the bottom of the brain is forced onto the top of the bony spinal column) — that can lead to death. Both type and level of response to increased pressure may vary with amount of pressure and damage, ranging from agitation, confusion, and chaos to little or no apparent response other than *coma*. Muscle weakness or difficulties with speech or vision may occur.

What is a *seizure* and what causes it?
A *seizure* is a sudden, random, abnormal electrical discharge from cerebral neurons that commonly results in involuntary muscle spasms (jerking), followed by sleep. Symptoms vary from only slight alteration of consciousness to a dramatic loss of consciousness. *Seizures* may result in slight facial tremors or staring spells, a cry, a fall, convulsions, incontinence, and amnesia for the seizure event.

Seizures may be caused by pressure on brain structures and neurons, the extra electrical activity in the brain that results from pressure and fluid imbalance, or both. Too much neurotransmission is another possible source (Stahl 2000). In this case, neurons are over-excited and fire when and where they should not. Some *seizures* are caused by scars that develop from cellular damage due to a previous injury. There are various types of *seizures*: generalized (grand mal), absence (petit mal), complex-partial, focal, psychomotor. Some seizures are a mixture of several types.

Penetrating injuries are associated with a higher incidence of post-traumatic *seizures* because they result in both skull fractures and brain wounds. (A *seizure* may also be the first sign of a brain tumor in otherwise symptom-free people.)

Two to five percent of all non-military brain injuries produce *seizures* within one week after injury (Slagle, in Miller, 1993). These early seizures do not lead to lifetime epilepsy as frequently as those that occur later, but psychiatric problems are often associated with *seizures* that occur within this first week. Risk factors include depressed skull fracture, focal brain injury with a *mass lesion* (large wound or hematoma), neurosurgical intervention, and relatively long duration of impaired consciousness.

What is a *cerebrovascular accident* (CVA) or *stroke?*
Stroke is another name for *cerebrovascular accident* (CVA). During a CVA, the brain's oxygen and blood supply is interrupted. After four to six minutes, neurons start to die. Nutrients and oxygen to the brain may be disrupted by:

- *Ischemic stroke* that occurs when plaque builds up and *occludes* (blocks) an artery.
- Pressure from an *aneurysm*, which is a pouch in the weakened blood vessel walls created by a piece of plaque.
- *Hemorrhage* resulting from the rupture of an *aneurism*.
- *Embolic stroke* that occurs when a blood clots breaks off and occludes an artery.

Brain damage from strokes may be localized or generalized. The kind of damage depends on which *neurons* have died and the location of the affected brain structures and systems. Damage in the *left hemisphere* usually affects verbal, analytic, and mathematical functions. Damage in the *right hemisphere* is likely to impair visual-spatial, musical, and some types of emotional functioning.

General effects can include problems similar to other brain injuries: fatigue, concentration, and memory problems, and emotional/behavior control problems, depending on the location of damage. Additionally, about half of all stroke survivors experience depression ranging from mild to severe, and nearly all experience grief.

What is a brain *tumor*?

A brain *tumor* is composed of brain or other tissue that grows too rapidly and forms an abnormal mass that takes up space and crowds or infiltrates normal brain tissue. *Tumors* may be *malignant* (cancerous) or *benign* (non-cancerous) and may develop from the brain itself (primary) or as a result of cancer that has spread from other parts of the body (secondary). *Tumors* may start out benign but with time may become malignant and *metastasize* (spread).

The kind and extent of damage depends on the location of the tumor, with hemispheric effects similar to those caused by a *stroke* and general effects similar to other brain injuries.

In most cases, a person's type of behavior and lifestyle do not cause a brain *tumor.* Tumors develop independently, without inflammation.

Brain 103: Treatments and Tests

How are brain injuries treated?

When a brain-injury survivor first arrives at the hospital, he is stabilized. Many different treatments and equipment may be used. Depending upon the kind of injury, the following may occur to stabilize the survivor:

- Bleeding is stopped using direct pressure, stitches, and/or a head dressing.
- Breathing is maintained, using a machine called a *ventilator* if necessary.
- Intracranial pressure is monitored and increased pressure is prevented and/or controlled. Physical stabilization is attempted by elevating the head and positioning the body to maintain alignment of the neck. Intake of fluids may be restricted to try to prevent the build-up of fluid pressure in the brain. Medication and/or surgery may be necessary.
- Infections are prevented and/or treated.
- Large blood clots in the brain are removed or prevented.
- Pain is controlled.
- Assistance is provided, if needed, for feeding, moving, bowel, bladder, and skin care.
- Medications may be required (as discussed below).
- Surgery may be required to relieve causes of increased cranial pressure, remove blood clots that place pressure on the brain, or remove skull fragments or massive tissue injury.

Preventive care is also given:

- **To prevent blood clots in the legs** from inactivity: special stockings may be fitted, such as anti-embolism stockings like TEDS (long, white elastic stockings) or sequential compression stockings like Kendalls (plastic leg-wraps that inflate and deflate to help prevent blood pooling in the legs).
- **To prevent bed sores** and assist with skin care: the skin is kept dry and clean, the survivor is repositioned on a regular schedule, and special pads and mattresses may be used.

- **To assist with moving:** splints and *range-of-motion* exercises may be prescribed to prevent *contractures* (tight muscles and joints).

Medications may include:
- **Diuretics** to reduce brain swelling by decreasing the amount of water in the body.
- **Steroids** to decrease brain tissue swelling.
- **Barbiturates** to induce a coma to put the brain at rest. This slow down the brain's reaction to the injury to avoid some of the damage if the intracranial pressure is very high and hard to control.
- **Anticonvulsants** to prevent seizures.
- **Analgesics** to control pain.

Surgical procedures to remove skull fragments or massive tissue injury may include:
- **Craniotomy or craniectomy** to open the skull to relieve the increased intracranial pressure.
- **Burr hole** made into the skull to remove a blood clot that is putting pressure on the brain.
- **Bone flap removal** from the skull to release pressure.
- **Ventriculostomy** to monitor intracerebral pressure. A small tube (called a *ventricular shunt* or *drain*) is inserted into the brain through a small hole in the skull to drain off extra fluid and to monitor *intracranial pressure* (ICP; pressure inside the head).
- **Other surgeries with the prefix "ventri-"** may be performed to view the *ventricles* (the cavities located in the cerebral hemispheres) using an endoscope or as part of special X-ray procedures.

What is the purpose of the devices used in intensive care?

The *monitor screen* displays vital signs, such as heart rate, breathing, blood pressure, and *intracranial pressure* (ICP).

The *ECG* or *EKG (electrocardiogram)* records the electrical activity of his heart through electrodes attached to his chest.

An *intravenous catheter (IV)* is inserted into an arm or leg vein to administer fluid, nutrients, and medicine.

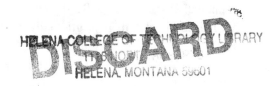

An *endotracheal tube* may be inserted through his nose or mouth, into his *trachea* (windpipe), or into his lungs to aid breathing, coughing up phlegm, and suctioning the lungs.

A *nasogastric tube (NG),* inserted through his nose, transports liquids and medications directly into his stomach.

A *Foley catheter* is a tube inserted into the bladder to drain and measure urine.

What do the neurological machines measure and why are they used?
Developed in the 1930s, the *electroencephalogram (EEG)* is one of the oldest neurological tests. The EEG measures electrical activity in different parts of the brain through electrodes placed at certain sites on the surface of the skull. Brain waves are graphed and analyzed to determine areas of slowed or irregular activity that may indicate the site and kind of brain abnormalities, e.g., focal brain damage and seizure activity.

The *quantitative EEG (QEEG)* uses a computer to analyze the brain's electrical activity. Brain areas are mapped using waveforms that represent the brain's electrical activity when repeatedly presented with a sensory stimulus.

An *X-ray* is a high-energy electromagnetic wave that penetrates most solid matter to produce a two-dimensional picture in five to thirty minutes. Typically used to look for bone fractures, an X-ray may miss small lesions and cannot detect biochemical disturbances in the brain.

The *CT scan (*the older term for this test is *CAT scan)* uses computerized axial tomography to produce a series of cross-sectional views of the brain or other body parts from *X-ray* information taken during a diagnostic scan that usually lasts 30-60 minutes. It can show more precise location of normal/abnormal structures than conventional x-rays, but is rapidly being replaced by newer technologies.

The *MRI (Magnetic Resonance Imaging)* uses radiofrequency pulse waves to take a sequence of detailed images while the brain processes specific information. MRI machines are shaped like long tubes. Although the scan is noisy, it is painless and produces a diagnostic picture in about 60 minutes. Because the MRI shows certain small brain structures and abnormalities in detail, it is gradually replacing the CT scan for some diagnostic purposes, although neither can identify microscopic lesions like diffuse axonal injuries or neurochemical changes that create functional impairments.

Functional MRI (fMRI) is a relatively new procedure that measures tiny metabolic changes that occur in an active part of the brain. It can map which part of the brain handles critical functions. fMRI also can help to assess the effects of stroke, trauma, and degenerative diseases; monitor growth and function of brain tumors; and guide plans for surgery, radiation, or other treatments.

Positron emission tomography (PET) scans provide a colored visual display of brain structure and function using a radioactive glucose substance. The degree of activity in particular brain areas is measured by the speed of glucose utilization; the more active areas of the brain metabolize glucose more rapidly. While PET scans can provide important information, they are expensive and not widely available.

Single photon emission computer tomography (SPECT) uses a readily available and more economic tracer compound to assess regional cerebral blood flow. *SPECTs* more accurately show focal cerebral lesions than either CT and/or MRI scans. Like the PET, these are expensive tests and not widely available.

Angiogram is a series of X-ray pictures of blood vessels that are taken in rapid sequence after an injection of a special dye into a blood vessel. Taking one to three hours, this test shows damage to veins, arteries, and various tissues.

In what other ways is neurological function measured and why?

Long before the sophisticated machines of the late 20th century were developed, neurologists of the late 19th and early 20th centuries accurately diagnosed brain dysfunction by skillfully using just their eyes, ears, hands, and minds. Let's see how the human touch assesses survivors.

Neurological exams: A series of clinical tests that examine the functioning of a person's nervous system by assessing his sensory, motor, and mental responses to a series of questions and commands given by a *neurologist*. The assessment includes a physical exam, ranges from simple to complex, and can take anywhere from a few minutes to an hour or more. Reflexes, voluntary behaviors, and cranial nerves are among the areas tested. Some examples of commands and questions included are "Close your eyes and touch your nose with your index finger." "Can you wiggle your toes?" "What day is it?"

Neuropsychological assessment: Some clinicians today feel strongly that for rehabilitation a neuropsychological testing evaluation is the most objective diagnostic tool and provides the greatest information. The advantage of these clinical tests is that they measure functional ability, which is not necessarily tied directly to the physical structures that the machines evaluate. They include detailed evaluation of a person's cognitive, emotional, and behavioral functioning by a *neuropsychologist* who uses the results from a battery of *standardized* tests, and other information, such as history and records, interview, and observation to develop a profile. Because TBI effects are so variable, many functions must be assessed for a complete picture. Taking up to 12 hours to complete, these extensive tests may be spread over several days. They measure brain-behavior relationships in attention, concentration, problem-solving, verbal and spatial reasoning, language, memory, intellectual level, motor, sensory-perceptual, and basic personality. The exam may be repeated periodically to monitor recovery and assess for permanent damage.

What is the purpose of all the tests? Why are they repeated?
There are medical and legal purposes for the tests.

Medically: the tests can measure changes in condition to update treatment plans and adjust different therapy regimens.

Legally: the tests may provide evidence for use in a lawsuit. Tests may be repeated because someone else wants to evaluate your survivor's condition. If lawyers are involved, expect that your survivor will see several doctors who will provide expert opinions for courtroom use and that each one may want to obtain his or her own findings.

Personal experience. For years following my 1976 accident — because there was no settlement until the early 1980s — I remember being retested at least four times with the same instruments by the opposing insurance companies' doctors, depending on which attorney remained on the case. While the scores varied, there was a consistent discrepancy between my performance and verbal IQ tests — which I later learned indicated brain damage. I surely wish someone had told me that I had a brain injury, so I would think I was still smart instead of a failure!

Sometimes the process can be amusing: Until the case was settled, I was asked to submit to the MMPI (Minnesota Multiphasic Personality Inventory) 13 times! Back in the early 1980s, when the medications changed, so did my craziness! Dare I divulge that the profile varied, depending on my medication, mood, and motivation? It became a game for me to see if I could produce a desired profile.

Ask for the purpose of the evaluations before submitting your loved one to them. And be sure to ask if prior results can be used rather than re-testing — the doctors may not know that the tests were previously done.

Why are the tests so difficult and time-consuming?

The tests are designed to be comprehensive, but there is controversy today whether a lengthy battery of tests provides more useful information than a shorter exam. Issues of fatigue, motivation, reliability, culture, and effects from chronic pain or medication need consideration. The longer tests may be more useful because they aid understanding of the survivor's strengths and deficits, guide treatment goals, and help predict recovery and functional capability.

> However patient survivors, family members, and professionals try to be, they need to double it and double it again. The recovery time-line is slow. Seeds sown now may flower years from now.
> — Wanda Windsor

Brain 104: Recovery/Rewiring Questions

Can the brain ever recover its functions?

Research in this area is very positive. Validating my "Use it or lose it!" motto, an increasing number of both laboratory and clinical studies demonstrate that recovery "may be dependent on some combination of drug therapy and rehabilitation or physical training," rather than the previously believed-in "spontaneous healing" and/or pharmacological treatment (Stein, Brailowsky, & Will, 1995).

Exciting news! Recent clinical trials with robotic devices add to the large body of evidence that suggests that repeated practice with an impaired limb can foster changes in the brain. This means that the robotic device can help the brain to form new connections between neurons or strengthen existing ones. For survivors, the result is that movement therapy helps the brain to use other nearby or non-damaged neurons to complete a movement! (Schaffer, 2007). See *Brain Injury Rewiring for Survivors* to learn more about brain repair and recovery and the goals of rehabilitation.

How can rehabilitation help my survivor?
Research has shown a strong relationship between the amount of quality intervention that a survivor engages in and the resulting positive functional change. Observe what occurs in his therapy — if it doesn't meet your expectations, share your concerns and ask questions. Then, if you are still not satisfied, find a different place!

Starting rehabilitation (rehab) is typically a hopeful time. Changing the focus from stabilization to improvement provides optimism from all concerned. Additionally, when therapy starts, there is often an enhanced ability to get along with people that occurs at the same time. This may be partly due to a survivor's increased self-confidence that results from improvement in functioning and greater independence. Surely, the support and acknowledgment by the rehab staff that the symptoms are real and problems not "all in his head" plays a big role. Healing requires time and everyone's best efforts!

What behaviors can we expect from him during the rehab process?
First, realize that in all recovery from brain injury, behavior is unpredictable although some behaviors are common. The most important thing to realize is that nothing about your survivor is the same as it was and probably never will be. Second, because of the normalcy of his appearance and what are often not easily recognizable problems, your survivor himself is confused about why he doesn't act like himself and

finds previously easily accomplished tasks difficult or impossible to perform. His diffuse brain damage isn't visible and he is as mystified and frustrated as you are! It is not uncommon to survive even a moderate brain injury and appear normal. In some ways, this normalcy brings with it more problems — your survivor's expectations of himself and other people's expectations of him — than if he appeared injured.

Slowness and executive function. Vocabulary and general information are largely not disrupted by brain damage and are about the same as pre-injury intelligence. However, slowness will be noticeable even if tests show that his pre-injury intelligence remains. Executive function — the ability to problem-solve — can be measured in many ways, however remember that the results are influenced by several factors.

- **Testing situations** are structured — and often require an exact response. Many survivors can pay attention, concentrate, and perform well in structured settings, yet find it difficult to respond to open-ended questions and in informal arrangements where it's a challenge to concentrate. In social settings, speed and efficiency of response often indicate whether someone is "with it."
- **Emotional factors** like anxiety, depression, and the psychological trauma of the injury itself affect general socializing and often impair memory, concentration, and thinking.
- **Physical factors** like pain, fatigue, sensitivity to noise and/or light, change in medications/dosages, and dietary/water intake could even stupefy Einstein!

Memory differences can be obvious. Here's a typical situation: "How can my son recite all the presidents' names this morning yet not remember the sports story I told him last night? I'm confused — he used to love sports — what is going on?" He may still love sports, and there are several reasons for this seeming difference.

- In most cases of brain injury, memory for information learned before the injury is mostly intact compared to new learning and retention — he can remember what he studied years before in high school but not what he heard today.

- Because brain injuries cause fatigue, which is a major factor in retention problems, most survivors perform best in the mornings when they are fresh.
- Perhaps his ability to learn by listening is different now. Before the injury, he may have learned easily by listening to new information. Now he may need different or several avenues to learn — seeing, doing, saying, and hearing — to master new information.

Moodiness is a result of the massive shock to body and brain and is troublesome for all. Your survivor may be as surprised and dismayed by his reactions as others are. Because his injured brain is less able to control emotional expression, he may seem angry, unhappy, tearful, or apathetic much of the time.

Many possible explanations can account for his responses. Besides physical shock, he likely feels grief, sorrow, and despair about his devastating loss. And, regardless of the depth of his awareness, he is not where he wants to be and is probably afraid of what will happen in the future. His cognitive abilities, such as reasoning, may be less able to regulate emotional reactions — difficulty in processing information leads to misperceptions and misinterpretations.

Superimposed on all of these reasons are the same internal and external physical factors that affect his cognitive abilities: nutrition, medication, sleep status, time-of-day, weather, room environment, phone calls, and/or visitors, even his favorite sports team's performance. Whew!

Are his responses due to the injury or emotional?

Does it matter? This is like asking the chicken-and-egg question — which came first! They're intertwined — a complex relationship exists between physical brain damage and reaction to the damage. Help everyone to cope better by remembering that studies show that actual physical injury is the cause of most, if not all, of the abnormal behaviors.

> Anger is a symptom, a way of cloaking and expressing feelings too awful to express directly — hurt, bitterness, grief, and most of all, fear.
> — Joan Rivers

As your survivor learns about how the injury affects his brain and personality, he can work to learn to control his behavior because of *neural plasticity* — the brain's ability to change and repair itself. Two of my favorite sayings on this topic are

- Knowledge is power.
- Behavior change precedes attitude change.

Consider, too, that anger is a common response and is a good sign — it means your survivor is fighting! You will cope better — and can help him to cope better — knowing that as he improves, he will gradually be less unhappy, angry, and moody. There is hope! See Chapter 6, Emotional Rewiring, to learn more.

What role do family and friends play?

Whether optimistic or pessimistic, the response of family and friends is critical to recovery. Criticism and negative emotions such as blame, although possibly due to

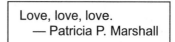

Love, love, love.
— Patricia P. Marshall

anxiety about your survivor, can create feelings of guilt, frustration, and even more of a sense of incompetence because your survivor is not the same as he was — and knows it! Common and natural attitudes such as shock, guilt, denial, confusion, resentment, and rejection strongly and negatively influence recovery — no kidding! Remember that positive communication helps a great deal. You are his connection to the rest of the world. His interactions with himself and others reflect yours — positive or negative.

Personal experience. Most of my family members were unable to be as involved or provide the support that I needed, due to physical and/or emotional distance. But they did the best they could. I was not totally abandoned and a close friend — really, my first angel — took over the key-person role. In my family's defense, little was known about TBI during the 1970s, and resources were scarce, so my family did not know what I needed or where to go for assistance.

Research tells us that the best outcome is achieved by those survivors whose families are involved with the treatment team — supportive and accepting of both him and his team — and realistic about his deficits and outcome. Luckily, rehabilitation is still possible when there are few obvious family resources beyond good genes, as my story shows. Although studies demonstrate the importance of family to recovery, I am testimony that little beyond a gifted gene pool, strong family values, and an angelic friend are truly required — did I mention the hand of God?

To use the mountain-climbing analogy again: everyone's climb up the mountain will be easier if you focus your energies on helping your survivor learn how to compensate for either his or his equipment's limitations and how to modify his environment — remove or reduce obstacles — rather than hoping either he or his equipment will become like it used to be. Remember The Golden Rule — "Do unto others…"

> Expect people to be better than they are; it helps them to become better. But don't be disappointed when they are not; it helps them to keep trying.
> — Merry Browne

Sometimes — or maybe often — you will find it difficult to feel positive and supportive. Of course! Your family "system" was injured, too. It has been said that the family members are the true victims of brain injury. Individual family members, especially the parents or spouses as well as the family system as a whole, are affected by the injury. Family dynamics are changed; roles and expectations need to be altered to fit with the new system. Therefore, it is important that your family receives help to adjust to the survivor and, as much as possible, to rehabilitate him within the context of the family.

During those times when you feel overloaded by all his needs, take time for yourself. Change your scenery by leaving the area — this helps you avoid saying or doing anything you'll regret. Give him a break and give yourself a break. A change can be refreshing to everyone.

Where can our family get help to adjust?
Psychotherapy can help all of you adapt to the changes in the family dynamics. Individual members will find that a counseling session is a safe place to express emotions that they may be unaware of or embarrassed to express.

Family therapy is a place to vent, to problem-solve, and to develop solutions. Family members can develop a plan together that considers everyone's needs and incorporates your survivor into the family system. You and your family can return to therapy to analyze what isn't working, reformulate possible solutions, and agree to try again. It can be a place where the needs of the family as a functional unit are placed above the needs of any member — injured or not. For these reasons, family therapy is recommended.

What can we do to help when he appears slow and unmotivated?

- Ask him what he needs. If he gives a vague answer like "I don't know," offer a few suggestions: sleep, nutrition, exercise, change of scenery or activity or topic.

> I need to take care of myself first or I can't take care of anyone else.
> — Bill Mate, Methodist minister

- Wait! Give him time to process. Ask him to tell you when he's ready.
- Keep trying to help find activities that engage him.
- Remind him of his goals.
- Role-model and explore a wide range of interests with him
- Help him create the habit of success at small tasks so he attempts other more complex projects.

> The healthy, the strong individual, is the one who asks for help when he needs it whether he's got an abscess on his knee or in his soul.
> — Rona Barrett

- Don't patronize or criticize — do NOT say or imply that he could do better if he tried or that he's lazy, etc.
- Invite him to join you in your activities.
- Accompany him to local brain-injury foundation meetings.
- Remember that what works today may not work tomorrow.
- Establish — with the help of professionals — what is and is not possible for him to change. His permanent neurological and physical impairments will dictate the best course of action and whether to compensate or substitute for an area of deficit.

What kind of home environment improves healing?

Major gains result from sensory-rich settings, even after the brain has supposedly finished healing. A home that is full of books and music provides outlets and opportunities for learning and creative expression. Stimulating and positive interaction with others gives survivors the best chance of recovery. Be sure that plenty of green plants surround him, too. The more oxygen, the better! Time with Nature is vital.

Laboratory research demonstrates that rodents allowed to play with toys develop more *dendritic* connections — contacts between *neurons* in the brain — than rodents raised in empty cages. Further studies found that even a daily two-hour enrichment period caused improvement in

> The greatest good you can do for another is not just to share your riches but to reveal to him his own.
> — Benjamin Disraeli

learning ability, regardless of age of animal or time since injury. The same is true for humans. Practicing mental processing and physical activity/exercise helps people develop and maintain competence in a wide range of activities as they age.

Work with a therapist to devise a program. Like a school classroom, the best environment provides structure, consistency, repetition of daily activities, success, and lots of rewards for both performance and effort.

> Take pleasure in the beauty and the wonders of nature.
> — Ann Landers

Where should we focus our energies? On physical or mental problems?

Consider the interaction and interrelation-ship of all the parts of our brain. Each part affects other areas. Many times resolving one problem significantly impacts other problems. For example, if dizziness is

> The work will teach you how to do it.
> — Estonian Proverb

eliminated and postural balance reestablished, then concentration and attention can get better, which leads to improved thinking skills. If the world is spinning, no one is able to pay attention to any part of it until the spinning stops.

What are his chances for recovery?

No one knows. Doctors are often asked to predict the future — "What's going to happen?" Yet, with brain injury the outcome is unpredictable. Medical professionals don't want to promise too much and create false hope that harms everyone, so a realistic outlook is very important. It is as great a disservice to a survivor and his family to be overly optimistic as to be overly pessimistic.

Unrealistic expectations, either too high or too low, can harm everyone. Consider how it would be if loved ones were told, "He'll be as good as new. Just give it time" and then — despite everyone's best efforts — he didn't recover his lost skills. The emotional turmoil for everyone concerned could be devastating, and what skills he did regain would be diminished in relation to what was lost.

> Trust yourself. You know more than you think you do.
> — Benjamin Spock

Christine Baser, PhD says, "The survivor may feel like a disappointment to others because he 'failed' and fell short of his expected recovery. I tell people to keep hope for the best outcome, but be prepared for problems or setbacks. This prevents people from limiting potential but also minimizes despair."

Keep in mind that doctors base their predictions on research results, so the particular studies they read affect their opinion. For example, some may pay more attention to studies that relate expected outcome to severity of injury, while others prefer to consider studies that suggest that recovery can be predicted from pre-injury factors such as personality traits.

> If the only tool you have is a hammer, you tend to see every problem as a nail.
> — Abraham Maslow

Because I believe that willpower and hard work determine outcome, I seek studies that investigate what can be done rather than what cannot. I am currently very excited about the new research regarding neuroplasticity, tissue implants, and regeneration of brain tissue. With the aging population and more interest in brain research, we can expect good news that will assist all of us who seek improved rewiring!

Remember that recovery depends on many factors: the survivor's personality, lifestyle, work ethic, general health behaviors like tobacco/alcohol/substance use and exercise/fitness, location and extent of brain damage, social support system, kind and amount of rehabilitation, divine intervention — and luck and hard work!

How can we all survive this journey to recovery?

Keep the faith and stay calm. Remember that your survivor is doing the best he can at any given time. Your support enables him to fully use all his capabilities to cope with the present situation instead of having to use part of his brain to block out negative feedback.

> Patience and faith is what the sea teaches... patience and faith.
> — Anne Morrow Lindbergh

So put the best light on everything — seek out the positive in everyone. We all need to feel we are liked, appreciated, and loved for who we are now. To think and act as though we and everyone else is okay — lovable and accepted, despite flaws or limitations — is the basis for positive interaction. We can all make it up this mountain!

Summary

- Ask him what he needs. If he says, "I don't know," suggest sleep, food or drink, exercise, change of scenery or activity or topic.
- Wait and give him time to process. Ask him when he's ready.
- Keep trying to help find activities that engage him.

> Keep hope for the best outcome, but be prepared for problems or setbacks to prevent limiting his potential and minimizing despair.
> — C. Baser

- Encourage his participation in rehab and remind him of his goals.
- Role model and explore a wide range of interests with him.
- Help him create the habit of success at small tasks so he attempts other more complex projects.
- Don't patronize or criticize. Do not say or imply that he could do better if he tried or that he's lazy, etc.
- Invite him to join you in your activities. Accompany him to local brain injury foundation meetings.

- Remember that what works today may not work tomorrow.
- Establish — with the help of professionals — what is and is not possible for your survivor to change. What he can change will dictate the best course of action and whether to compensate or substitute for a deficit area.
- Surround him with stimulating and positive people.
- Create a healthy environment with natural light, plants, and pets.
- Ensure he spends time every day with Nature.
- Work with a therapist to devise a recovery program for your survivor and your family.
- Consider the interrelationship of all the parts of our brains — often resolving one problem significantly impacts and improves other problems.

4

Spiritual Rewiring: Healing Hearts with Prayer and the Arts

When you have a disease, do not try to cure it.
Find your center, and you will be healed.
— Taoist proverb

Healing on the spiritual level precedes and affects everything else. This chapter explores how you can heal your spirit as well as help your survivor on his journey to heal his. When people feel centered and in sync, they are receptive to working on challenging emotional issues and better able to implement suggested strategies. Through the use of prayer and the arts, especially music, we learn how to find our center and help our survivor to find his. The topics include:

- Your sonic environment and how to create one that heals.
- How to chart your heart.
- The Mozart Effect: what music can do.
- Suggested composers and tunes to suit our various moods.
- Spiritual healing practices: ancient and current healing rituals.
- Other expressive arts: visual, auditory, and physical arts.
- Receptive arts: listening, reading, enjoying theater, dance, and nature.

Introduction

"Sure, I'd like to believe the Taoist proverb that tells me we'll be healed after we find our centers, but I'm really too busy right now to do that. It seems all I do is drive my survivor to medical appointments to try to find answers to all my questions about how to repair his injury. I'm far too tired to think about myself and how to find my center. Besides, I'm fine — it's him I'm worried about."

"We've seen so many medical people and tried everything everybody suggested — and yet nothing seems to make much of a difference. In fact, he seems to be getting worse! Now he's angry from the instant he awakens, doesn't want to do anything or be with anyone, and isolates himself in his room, playing his loud and discordant music all day. The sounds are the same ones he liked before his injury, but now he acts so differently! His former joy and playfulness have disappeared. Basically, he just seems so out of sync with life and himself."

Does this sound familiar? And are you actually "fine"?

You know that his brain was traumatized and heard that it'll take time for him to recover — that time will heal him. Professionals may have also told you there's nothing you can do except follow their directives for him to take his medicines and do his therapies.

You want to believe this — but he's driving you and other loved ones crazier the longer this recovery stage goes on. Perhaps the rest of the family says they love him but find lots of reasons to avoid him and stay away from home. They may say they're "fine," too, but seem angry and accuse you of loving him more than them. Maybe nobody is "fine." How about at least trying this centering thing? You've tried everything else!

Do we really need to change our home environment?

Yes — because after the injury, nothing is the same anymore. While it's true that routine is comfortable and helps maintain a sense of normalcy, when one member changes, so do the dynamics of the home. Keeping some things the way they were helps the transition. However, it is likely that the former sonic environment no longer works for the survivor and therefore for no one else in the family either, so changing that is a good place to start.

How will music and sounds help to create a healing atmosphere?
Sound and vibration surround us every minute of our lives. Healthy rewiring depends upon therapeutic sounds and music. Don't we want our sonic environment to heal rather than harm?

"By paying close attention to the pulse, pace, and pattern of music, you can create a sonic diet to keep you energized, refreshed, and relaxed throughout the changing seasons of your life" (Campbell, 1997).

How do I change our sonic environment?
First — you, your survivor, and other loved ones need to observe how music affects you by charting your hearts. Then you can make changes.

Charting your heart is a way to discover which music and sounds create the most therapeutic environment for you and your family, based upon what your bodies, minds, and spirits reveal. Music is selected based upon the desired energy state and/or activity. For example, music for eating will differ from that for physical tasks. It will also vary depending upon the time of day. See Chapter 4 in *Brain Injury Rewiring for Survivors* for directions on how to chart your hearts, then do it for all family members!

Music

Music is our original language. Supporting the theory that human beings communicated primarily with sound or tone before speech is a mid-1990s discovery of the world's oldest musical instrument, a bone flute from 43,000 to 82,000 years ago (Campbell, 1997).

> Music sets up a certain vibration, which unquestioningly results in a physical reaction. Eventually the proper vibration for every person will be found and utilized.
> — George Gershwin

Healing and protecting people with sound and music also dates back to ancient civilizations. People believed that higher powers or spirits ruled all of life, whether that involved the elements or other tribes. Everything was caused — and could therefore be resolved — by the spirits (Campbell, 1997).

To invoke spirits to heal and protect was the role of the shaman, who acted as the bridge to the other world using direct power from the divine source. We may not still believe in shamans, but music is still a powerful source of healing energy we can use to help our survivor and ourselves during recovery.

The Mozart Effect

Ever hear of the Mozart Effect? It is the impact of the vibrations of music and other environmental sounds upon our skin and our bones that influence body and brain functions. We make a connection to the deeper rhythms of life that can lead to self-generated healing (Campbell, 1997).

> In terms of healing, The Mozart Effect extends far beyond the sound itself...You determine the final impact. You are an active conductor and participant in the process of orchestrating health.
> — Don Campbell

Music affects heartbeat, breathing, and digestion.

Our heart rate reflects the musical variables of tempo, frequency, and volume, slowing down or speeding up to match the rhythm of the sound. So it is with respiration — breathing is rhythmic. Lower heart rate and breathing rate lead to a healthy and well-functioning body. Food digests better when we are calm. Consider why many eating and drinking establishments play loud and fast music — don't we eat and drink more?

Music affects blood pressure and body temperature.

The faster the music, the faster the heart beats, which in turn increases the pressure of the blood on the wall of the blood vessels. Calming the beating heart reduces blood pressure, slows circulation, and cools the heating system. Speed up to warm up, slow down to cool down.

Music can regulate brain waves.

Ever hear of *beta* or *alpha waves*? When we focus on our daily activities and when we feel strong negative emotions, our brains produce *beta waves* that vibrate between 14 and 20 Hertz. (Brain waves are measured in a unit of frequency called Hertz, which is equal to one cycle per second). *Alpha waves* oscillate between 8 and 13 Hertz and correspond to a state of calm alertness and general well-being. Music with a 60-beats-per-minute pace — like Mozart's — and practices like yoga and meditation can alter brain waves from *beta* to *alpha*.

If you or your survivor feel dreamy or emotionally scattered, you can play a little Mozart, Baroque, or New Age music to steady your conscious awareness and organize and refocus your minds. On the other hand, when you're stuck in a rut, jazz, or other improvisational sounds release logical constraints to send you dreaming and creating.

Music and sound can regulate stress-related hormones.
Consider our fight-or-flight response to an emergency. Our hearts beat faster, blood pressure increases, palms sweat, and digestion slows — demonstrating how our emotional states influence all body systems. These physiological changes are an attempt to restore balance after an intrusion by what is perceived as a stressor. To ward off the intruder or flee, our muscles need additional fuel, so the adrenal gland releases stress-related hormones like adrenaline and cortisol to mobilize these changes.

To be able to respond quickly to danger is vital. However, to remain in this state of readiness for extended periods depletes our resources and exhausts our adrenals. Listeners who chose their own relaxing music showed up to a 25% decrease in cortisol level. Listening to calming music during stressful, but not dangerous, times can slow our bodily systems, thus helping us save our resources for times of immediate danger.

Music can increase endorphin levels and boost immune function.
Do you know why you feel better when you hear music played? Endorphins — our natural opiates or painkillers — are released by the pituitary gland in the brain when music stimulates electrical activity.

Music, singing, chanting, and vocalizations also increase circulation and oxygenate cells, which is important for health. Insufficient blood oxygen is a major causative factor of immune deficiency and degenerative disease. Listening to music for just fifteen minutes can increase levels of interleukin-1 (a substance that promotes good immune function) in the blood by 12% to 14% and elevate levels of T-cells (lymphocytes that boost immunity to disease).

Music improves body movement and reduces muscle tension.
Ever wonder why your body naturally moves to music? Sound and vibration influence muscle strength, flexibility, and tone through the connections of the auditory nerve from our inner ear to all our muscles.

Stroke survivors who received rhythmic auditory stimulation for just thirty minutes a day for three weeks improved their cadence, stride, and foot placement — and the effects lasted!

Listening to a variety of musical selections ranging from New Age to popular to classical, participants with severe spastic conditions increased their range of movement in spines, hips, legs, and arms. Lower frequency (between 40 and 66 Hertz) music resonates in the lower body and higher frequency in the upper body. No wonder rehabilitation clinics play music during repetitive movement therapy! Research has found not only improved mood and motivation but also increased strength and coordination of exercisers in an aerobics class.

Music changes our perception of time and space.
We know we speed up or slow down in time with music. Did you ever notice how different your environment feels with fast versus slow music? Do you sense more space within the tones when slow music plays? Isn't fast music a crowd of sounds? Our sonic environment either confines us or liberates us. We can choose to create an environment that envelops us with more or less space. If we feel crowded by either time or space, we can select elegant music that enlarges our space, like Mozart's chamber music or ambient/New Age music like Steven Halperin's.

Music and sound mask unpleasant sounds and feelings.
It is no secret that noise upsets survivors' fragile wiring and creates systemic discord. Excessive noise can also raise blood pressure by as much as ten percent and may trigger the fight-or-flight response. *I still wince and run from that awful leaf blower noise!*

Just as disturbing tones disturb bone conduction, so do calming tones disguise, neutralize, and even repel harsh invasive environmental sounds.

Quiet Baroque music — and even humming — works to mask the sound and vibrations of dental drills. Remind your survivor to fight back with music the next time he feels violated by environmental sounds.

Music raises endurance.
Why did laborers sing while they worked? Songs with strong beats like "I've Been Workin' on the Railroad" promote strength.

Appropriate music can enhance the performance of any activity that demands stamina, especially those with their own cadence and rhythm, such as cycling and running. The power of music was demonstrated by a cyclist who increased his cycling performance by 25% when he listened to instrumental music while racing between California and New York, setting a world record pace of nine days, 23 hours, and 15 minutes.

Personal experience. I, too, can vouch for this effect after cycling from San Diego, California, to Cabo San Lucas, Mexico — about 1100 miles. Music provided good company to my pedal cadence, especially in the desert and on the mountain climbs!

Music can boost productivity, strengthen memory, and maximize ability to learn.
Just as it aids us physically, music strengthens mental abilities. By calming and organizing our minds, it enables us to study and learn effectively. When AT&T and DuPont used creative music programs for just six weeks, training times were cut by 50% and productivity increased between 17% and 19%!

> The power of music to integrate and cure... is quite fundamental. [It is the] profoundest non-chemical medication.
> — Oliver Sachs

Another study found that manuscript copyeditors who listened to light classical music increased their accuracy by 21% compared to a 2.4% increase for those who listened to a popular commercial radio format. Even an ambience of office noise is more conducive than silence, as shown by an 8.3% decrease in accuracy in those who edited in silence versus those who worked with the typical office noise.

Music enhances romantic feelings and unconscious receptivity to symbolism.

Think about movies with sensuous soundtracks. What kind of music evokes passion? A light and airy piece with a leisurely pace that also includes some tempestuous crescendos, like "Out of Africa," elicits romantic feelings in most people. Contrast that with frenetic pieces like "Riverdance," the Rolling Stones' "Honky Tonk Woman," and rap music, which typically don't evoke romantic feelings.

Now consider the symbolism of the harsh loud sounds of war movies contrasted with the sweet music of children's movies. Film directors use the auditory environment to tap the unconscious and enhance the mood created by what we see. Our receptivity to any message is so influenced by what we hear that a soundtrack can make or break a movie.

Music provides a safe expression of feelings and generates a sense of well-being.

What better way to express feelings — without harming anyone or anything — than through music? Whether we sing, play, or dance to it, music allows us to safely release and express our feelings of

> Without music, life is a journey through a desert.
> — Pat Conroy

sympathy, anger, fear, love, joy, sadness, or grief. It can also generate those same feelings and provoke us to action. Music also makes us feel good about ourselves, each other, and the world in general.

No matter the mood, we can find sounds that resonate with us. While those who grew up in the 1920s and 1930s sought refuge in familiar hymns and musicals to survive two world wars and the Depression, my 1960s generation found solace in Vietnam-era protest songs. Singers as diverse as Bob Dylan, Simon and Garfunkel, Joan Baez, and Judy Collins spoke for us and to us. More recently, Bruce Springsteen expressed both the anguish and triumph of 9/11 in "The Rising."

As both messenger and haven, music serves the same purpose today. With the electronic age simultaneously contracting and expanding our world, lyrics, volume, and rhythm can both distance us and touch us. New kinds of music offer varied choices to new generations who need new vehicles of expression just like all preceding generations. Although

the messenger may look unusual and bring a different message, music —
the medium — remains the same. The voice of music speaks for all the
people all the time.

How do I persuade my family to chart their hearts?
Chart your own heart first and play the music you need for various
activities. Your family may notice that you select different music based
upon your mood and needs, and may discuss it with you. If nobody
mentions it, you may want to talk about how an appropriate sonic
environment helps you focus on your activities, and then invite your
survivor and other family members to try it for themselves.

If your survivor declines to try charting his heart for any number of
reasons, firmly tell him you need him to do it because your sanity
depends upon it! If other family members likewise aren't inclined to do
it, ask them to do it because it would help the survivor.

While it is likely that your survivor's pre-injury music preferences
are no longer suitable/healthy for him and need to be reassessed, the
same holds true for all who reside in the home.

How do family music choices affect my survivor?
Remember that the discussion about sonic environment. Controlling your
survivor's environment is vital to his recovery because he is unable to
block out upsetting noise and music. Therefore, the kind of music played
in the home is central for successful rewiring as well as for harmony for
all!

How does noise or discordant music affect my survivor's brain?
Sudden loud noise — like sirens and
alarms — upsets delicate brain tissue that
is struggling to heal. Because his "sonic
screen" was damaged, when loud sound
invades his brain, he is unable to control

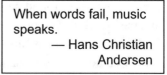

When words fail, music
speaks.
— Hans Christian
Andersen

the emotions it provokes — often anxiety, fear, and/or anger. Even if
your survivor plugs his ears, the damage has already begun. From a non-
verbal grimace to a cry, scream, or yell, he exhibits the pain caused by
upsetting sounds.

Harm can be minimized by an immediate exit, peaceful music, and a comforting hug. You can also help by shortening the "noise sentence" as much as possible to minimize damage — the less time he spends in a distressing place, the less time it takes to heal the wound.

Personal experience. Even thirty years after my injury, dissonant music and loud noise or talking — especially if sudden and nearby — disturb me. If I can't flee, I explain to the "offender" what the noise does to me — hopefully before I'm so disturbed that I'm abrasive. Most people respond kindly, although they usually say, "Just block it out." — If I could, I would!

If he's close to overload, what can I do — before his wiring shorts out?

To avoid distress, learn what sounds and noises overload his wires — usually anything sudden, loud, and discordant — then flee, fight, or negotiate. If escape isn't possible, remind him to drown out the offending noise with his choice of music or play something soothing. Then ask the one responsible for the sound or noise to either turn down the volume or turn the sound or noise off.

What can I do if he escaped too late — if his wiring shorted out?

Help him to ground himself (See *Brain Injury Rewiring for Survivors.*) Remind him to breathe deeply — this is a vital part of this process. Ask him if he wants any physical comforting. Allow him to remain grounded as long as he needs to regain a sense of peace and to re-arm himself to return to the world. How much he needs will depend on the degree of disturbance in his wiring.

After he grounds himself, it may be necessary to change the day's schedule so that he participates only in quiet activities with supportive people. Because of the insult to his wires, he will need time and a restful environment to heal the damage.

People who are unfamiliar with brain injury survivors will probably be perplexed and/or shocked by his response to noise. Don't focus on their response — just do whatever it takes to calm your survivor. Others will likely assist you with this goal — or at least not question you — if they know the consequences — screaming, shouting, hysterical crying, etc.

Music for various moods and workouts.
See *Brain Injury Rewiring for Survivors* for information about the best music for various situations. Below are some suggestions that are especially useful when your survivor's wires have been overloaded.

Special relaxation music:
The favorite calming music chosen by relaxation experts from different spas around the US were water sounds and panpipes (Cool. 1997).
- "Ascension" by Dean Evenson.
- "Canyon Trilogy, Vol. 5" by R. Carlos Nakai.
- "Dream Images" by Shardad Rohani.
- "Honorable Sky" by Peter Kater and R. Carlos Nakai.
- "The Inner Voyage" by Cristal Silence.
- "Mender of Hearts" by Crimson.
- "Nothing Above My Shoulders but the Evening" by Ray Lynch.
- "Pachelbel Canon & Ocean Sounds" by Anastasi.
- "Shadows" by Danny Wright.
- "Shepherd Moons" by Enya.
- "Skywatching" by Michael Gettel.
- "Tribal Winds" by various artists.

Other healing sounds (Carter):
- "Mind-Body Rhythms: Music for Healing" by Janalea Hoffman.
- "Music for the Mozart Effect."
- "Harmonic Resonance" by Emmy-winning composer Jim Oliver.
- "Inner Dance" by sound therapist Jeffrey Thompson.
- "Wind and Mountain" by Deuter.
- "Points of Light" by noted Russian composer Boris Mouashkin.

Spiritual Healing Practices

When we quiet our minds, we can hear the inner voices of our hearts. Then we can seek the Light both within and outside ourselves. We may begin to pray — even if we don't consider ourselves religious —

> Faith is the bird that sings when the dawn is still dark.
> — Tagore

whether we call it that or not. Desperate times call for desperate measures.

Because brain injury is an equal opportunity event, *Brain Injury Rewiring* readers come from all faith traditions, including no particular faith, as well as those who consider themselves spiritual but not religious. If you profess a faith, first look to it for ways that heal. See *Brain Injury Rewiring for Survivors* for a humorous story about someone who didn't hear God until it was too late.

If we don't feel a direct connection to God, then how do we pray?

Through the ages and in different faith traditions, people have sought and seek intermediaries to God, the unseen One. Various mediators are chosen, depending upon cultural and religious experiences. You may find something that resonates for you and/or your survivor.

> The reason there are many religions is the same reason there are many foods... Follow what grows best where you live.
> — Dalai Lama

Buddhists believe all beings may become saviors or teachers — *Buddha* means "teacher" — so they do not pray to or through a divine being. Rather, devotees seek an inner calmness and follow a Noble Path in their quest for nirvana. To transport them to a sacred healing state, they meditate on an image or listen to certain sounds and may use a mantra — often intoning the centering "om" sound to cleanse negative karmas (Craughwell, 1998).

Christians believe in the Trinity — God the Father, Son, and Holy Spirit. They pray to God, through Jesus, and in the Spirit. Jesus lived on this earth so He is the human connection and the Spirit is God within us. Our English word *spirit* comes from the Latin word for "breath," which combined the Greek and Hebrew words for "wind" and "breath." Spirit is everywhere, like breath and wind. Roman Catholics also pray to the Virgin Mary. Because she was an ordinary woman, coming to her to bridge the distance to God seems natural. Some Christians also pray to different saints — like St. Jude for "the impossible" for people with specific needs. Those who prefer dragon-slayers may pray to St. Michael, known as a warrior who fights the forces of evil and as one of the archangels, those angels closest to God. Some Biblical scholars believe that each human being has his or her own protecting angel (Metzger, 1993).

Hindus believe in an ultimate called Brahman, which is impersonal, and cannot be addressed in a personal way. However, Brahman is so pervasive that believers do not think about it as though it were separate — it is part of their being. It also manifests itself in many gods and goddesses, each of whom can receive prayers and devotion.

In the **Jewish and Islamic** traditions, prayer is directed to God as the heavenly Parent, and there are no intermediaries. Jesus and Mohammed are viewed as prophets — powerful recipients of God's word, but not divinities.

Native Americans believe "there's one God, Mother Earth, with the big man up at the top. It's all tied in" (Eugene Magee). Various symbolic objects are used to connect with the Divine, such as wooden totems and other effigies constructed from wood, cloth, and fur. Animated dolls and puppets are used by the Eskimos. Both to serve to connect to the Divine and for "demon control," thread crosses and yarn for God's eyes are favored by Tibetans and Mexicans (Barfield, 1998).

Shamanism is an ancient spiritual craft that employs the special skills and practices of a gifted person, the shaman, to nurture, supervise, and empower both individual and tribal healing. It is believed that as an intermediary between the visible and invisible worlds, the shaman transcends normal human consciousness to travel among different planes to guard individual and tribal psychic and ecological health and welfare.

Shamans, male or female, are known by various names throughout the world: medicine man or woman, witch doctor, sorcerer/ess, magician, witch, psychic, yogi, yogini, kahuna, seer, or medium (Phoenix & Arabeth, 1999).

What are some healing practices and rituals?

Ever since ancient times, humans around the world found inner peace and healing through various practices. Whether it was African dancing and drumming, Buddhist meditation, Tibetan singing bowls,

> I see God in every human being.
> — Mother Teresa

Christian laying-on of hands and anointing with oil, Hindu fasting and yoga, Moslem reading and study, Jewish prayers, or Native American sweat lodges, people sought spiritual enlightenment and health. See *Brain Injury Rewiring for Survivors* for descriptions of rituals and healing practices.

Expressive and Receptive Arts

Creating Music

We know that listening to music offers many benefits — playing it offers even more. Focusing on making music, rather than making appointments and making the injury better alters your mindset from negative to positive in just minutes! Imagine your moody survivor in an optimistic mood for a change.

"He used to love to play his guitar. Now he has time to find his soul again. Maybe I'll join him."

Even anticipating the opportunity to play works wonders. Reminding yourselves that after you do what you have to do, you can do what you want to do is guaranteed to improve everyone's outlook for the whole day! How about brainstorming about what you'll play as you await an appointment rather than wasting time just sitting? Rewarding yourselves with music also elevates the role it plays in your lives.

Playing musical instruments or singing — either alone or with others — not only provides a creative physical and emotional release but also raises intellectual abilities (Campbell, 1997).

Playing with another family member or friend increases enjoyment. Besides the social interaction, making music as a member of a group fosters a sense of belonging that survivors don't often experience.

Many community groups that provide a variety of musical opportunities at different skill levels await you and your survivor. Explore offerings at your local community college, city recreation department, public school adult education, and houses of worship.

What can you do to encourage a survivor's pursuit of creative arts?
Help him select appropriate background music. Remind him to follow his heart and his dream. Ask him what art he likes. Join him!

If he doesn't feel inspired to create, visit art museums and galleries. Explore the local library and bookstores. Or just venture outside, maybe take a camera. He will see that he is still connected to the universe, just in a different way than before his injury.

If he says he's not creative, tell him that everyone is and that some people just experience it sooner than others. Encourage him to explore different artistic mediums to uncover favorites and that to try is to succeed.

If he asks how art can heal him, remind him that just like music, other arts naturally transport us somewhere else. The arts relax us and free our minds from worry, so our brains and bodies can heal.

And, as astounding as it seems, his brain injury can make creating art easier! While his new behavior may sometimes — often? — displease you, embarrass him, and annoy others around you, his lack of inhibition enables him to rediscover his natural curiosity — and himself!

Assess his mood to determine whether to suggest that he investigate something new — and possibly difficult — or if he needs the comfort of a safe — easily successful — activity. The answer helps you decide what to do. Maybe you will decide to join him!

Visual Arts

Whether we paint with sand like ancient healers or sculpt with modern plastic materials, working with art media can satisfy the urge to express a variety of emotions for anyone, regardless of talent.

> What art offers is space… breathing room for the spirit.
> — John Updike

Restoring emotional balance and a sense of meaning and order to life can result from simply freeing the mind to express itself.

Some examples are drawing, painting with acrylics or watercolors, sculpting with clay or plastic, making masks, photographing indoors or outdoors, sewing, knitting, or other needlecraft activities. Perhaps your computer is loaded with a drawing program. Any of these media can be temporary or permanent.

Photography

Perhaps invest in a digital camera now that the cost is more reasonable. Numerous settings offer opportunities to experiment, pictures are downloaded to the computer, your survivor chooses which ones to print, and taking pictures is free! Perhaps he'll be willing to take pictures "that aren't any good" if there is no cost, thus freeing him to play with the camera and have fun.

Creative Writing/Speaking

Self-expression through the act of writing or speaking is not only a cathartic healing experience achieved through a non-violent release of emotions but may also serve as a learning tool (See also Chapter 5.) Creating text on the computer works for several reasons: any physical weakness can be more easily overcome, the files are organized, and material can be easily altered.

Writing poetry seems to be a popular escape route for many people — especially when in pain — but crafting short stories or prose poetry can be equally effective. Your survivor may say, "My arm/hand doesn't work well. How can I write?" Tell him: "You can talk, right? Speak into a tape recorder — it's easier and works, too." Computer speech-recognition programs are also becoming more economical and user-friendly.

Theater Arts

Your survivor may say, "My arm/hand doesn't work well. How can I act?" Tell him: "Acting doesn't require two hands or two legs — just a mouth, and emotions, which you've got!" Acting is a wonderful way to escape his injury! And it's a social experience that's not disability-based. Improvisation is the perfect theater for survivors because there is no right way and it's based on spontaneous behavior. Readers' theater offers another creative outlet. An expressive voice is all that is needed as "players" read parts in plays to themselves and each other. Find readers' theater groups through local adult-education classes, city recreation centers, or bookstores.

Physical Arts

If your survivor loved physical activity before his injury, encourage him to explore creative movement now. Whether accompanied by music or alone, it provides an artistic outlet that requires only free space and an unfettered spirit.

Dancing can be free or structured; mobility is not a deterrent. Any rhythmic movement is cathartic and improves mood. Join him!

> Flowers always make people better, happier, and more helpful; they are sunshine, food, and medicine to the soul.
> — Luther Burbank

Gardening enriches bodies, minds, and spirits. See Chapter 10 for more information.

Receptive Arts

Another way for him to derive the healing benefits of art is to receive and appreciate the efforts of others. Listening, watching, reading, smelling, touching — and maybe even tasting — the beauty available through Nature and the creations of artists also invokes the healing process.

Summary

I hope that Spiritual Rewiring helps you and your survivor to heal your hearts as you explore various artistic mediums.

> Art is the triumph over chaos.
> — John Cheever

Join him in his pursuit of creative arts! I also hope that recreating yourselves through art leads to many enjoyable hours with new friends in a community that is focused on something greater than disability — imagine that! Your survivor will usually find acceptance because the focus is on the activity and what can be done rather than on the problems and limitations of a disability. And you don't need to do it alone.

No one path will transport everyone to creative nirvana. Just be receptive to new ideas, to others, to the healing powers — and explore what feels right. You and he can heal your hearts with prayer and the arts. You can play your own music. It's worked for many years. Enjoy!

- Change your home environment to work for him now.
- Chart your hearts.
- Play the music that's best for each of your activities.
- To avoid distress, learn what sounds and noises overload his wiring — usually anything sudden, loud, and discordant — then flee, fight, or negotiate.
- If escape isn't possible, remind him to drown out the offending noise with his choice of music.
- Help him to ground himself if he escapes noise too late.
- If you profess a faith, first look to it for ways that heal.
- Play music to gain even more benefits than listening.
- Explore other creative arts.

5

Cognitive Rewiring: Healing Minds with Activities and Games

Just fix my brain and I won't be crazy! — or dumb or lazy or inappropriate…
— Carolyn E. Dolen

Frustrated survivors, including yours, probably utter something like this every day. He's doing the best he can with a broken brain. Supported by recent research that shows brains can rewire after injury — with work — Chapter 3 discussed how the brain is originally wired. This chapter explores how to fix his wiring. We explore what to repair and how to rewire his brain, growing new cells and connections so he can cognitively connect again. We answer common questions about the thought process and offer strategies, suggestions, activities, and resources to improve communication skills. Topics include:

- Introduction: "dead" doesn't mean "gone"
- What is cognitive functioning? What needs to be fixed?
- What are typical cognitive problems and related problem areas?
- Can cognitive connections improve? When? How?
- Cognitive therapy with professionals: what and how.
- After rehab: strategies, games, tools, and computer programs.
- Activities/aids to improve cognitive functioning and teach skills.
- Cognitive connection: communication do's and don'ts.
- Rewiring activities: quiet and active, alone and with others.

Introduction

Before he reads *Brain Injury Rewiring for Survivors*, your survivor may argue that his brain can't be fixed. He may say that brain cells don't regrow, that he doesn't want to bother to try to repair something that can't be fixed, and that he just wants to be left alone. Don't listen to him!

As he'll read in *Brain Injury Rewiring for Survivors,* the previous scientific theory about the brain — that all cells were created at birth and new ones didn't grow later — is itself dead! Findings about new tissue growth — even in older brains — thankfully puts to rest that old thinking (Stein, Brailowsky, & Will, 1995).

Studies of older people's brains supported earlier work with animals: Adult brains sprout between 500 and 1000 new cells per day (Eriksson, 1998). This seems miniscule compared to a total of 70 million cells in the hippocampus — but it all adds up, right? Of special interest are two factors: the new cell growth occurred in the area of the brain called the hippocampus, which is involved in learning and memory, and the study involved older people with cancer. Imagine the number of new neurons in young and healthy humans!

Recent PET scan studies demonstrated that not only does the brain grow new cells but it also forms new networks to bypass the injured areas (Levine et al., 2002). Researchers also found that one side of the brain can be trained to compensate for impairment on the other side (Abdulla, 2001). These latest studies validated my long-held belief in our own power to heal — if we just do it!

How can you spur new growth? Create an interesting environment for him. We don't need research to prove that physical and mental activity and social contact enhances growth — and based on research with residents of nursing homes and animals, scientists think this is what occurs (Eriksson, 1998; Hamm et al., 1996).

In one study, moderately injured animals that recuperated in a complex environment not only performed significantly better than those who recovered in a standard setting, but also performed as well as animals not actually injured! In this study, different types of bedding and objects provided motor, olfactory, tactile, and visual stimulation to improve cognitive recovery after TBI (Hamm et al., 1996).

Beyond the utter logic of it, stimulating body, mind, and spirit leads to a rich life. Yay! Let's fix our brains!

Personal observation. *I am living proof that we can fix our brains — we can continue to improve — if we work at it!*

What is cognitive functioning? What needs to be fixed?

Cognitive functioning is the mental process by which we use and acquire knowledge. When this is damaged, the control center and its wiring need an overhaul, starting with any dysfunction in the visual-perceptual systems.

Because the brain directs the whole body, treating this central-thinking operation affects all other functions — behavioral, emotional, social, and even physical (Namerov, 1987; Vogenthaler, 1987; Ben-Yishay et al., 1987). And because the problem areas correspond to the functions that the brain supports, when thinking ability increases, overall health improves. In fact, researchers state that thinking deficits clearly overshadow physical deficits as the cause of handicaps in independent living and social and vocational re-entry into the community (Ben-Yishay et al., 1987). Scientists draw these conclusions from their studies:

- Damaged cognitive functioning — even subtle deficits, vague symptoms, and weak coping skills create problems that may be misdiagnosed as psychiatric (Ben-Yishay et al., 1987). This lends credence to my statement: *"Fix my brain and I won't act crazy."*
- Cognitive functioning will likely significantly diminish whenever a survivor is exposed to stress, or is depressed or anxious. Additionally, survivors exhibit emotional sensitivity to some psychological tests (Sbordone 1987).
- To the extent that inappropriate behavior is related to impaired thinking, so will it improve with better cognitive functioning (Askenasy, 1987).

What are likely cognitive problems?

Just about anything imaginable. The best overall descriptor is the term *executive function deficit*, meaning that there is an inability or reduced ability to plan, organize, direct, control, remember, and carry out plans and tasks, and accomplish business.

Someone exhibiting this may look normal, appear competent to others, be enthusiastic and be able to perform well on structured tasks — yet in reality is unable to follow through when things are more complex.

Why is this important?

Unrealistic expectations naturally follow when survivors present an appearance of being with it — when they actually are not. When what you see is not what you get, we're all in trouble! To make it even more interesting, this may or may not be readily visible — even to professionals. Regardless of the reason for this appearance, it can lead to fewer recommendations for rehabilitation services than are needed, which results in some painful — and avoidable — social and vocational failures.

What are some related problem areas?

Memory. It is well known that memory disturbances occur in all brain injuries regardless of severity — including so-called minor injuries. Memory deficits are complex: survivors show inconsistencies across skill areas, within a skill area, and over time. In short, they're unpredictable!

Typically, people involved with survivors find that their memory for well-learned, pre-injury information — past knowledge — is strong in contrast to their ability to learn and remember new material. Brain burps — difficulty remembering incidental information — may cause survivors to misplace items, miss appointments, and forget conversations, routes to familiar locations, and even daily grooming routines.

Personal experience. If I have not been somewhere in over a week — unless it's a place I've visited many times — I need to verbally review directions, write them down, and take them with me. When I'm going to a new place, I also grab my street guide after marking the appropriate pages. Because driving alone is challenging enough, I stop alongside the road to check my guide when I make a mistake, rather than looking while navigating freeway traffic and construction — I hope this reassures my fellow travelers!

By the way, I don't get lost. Any deviation is an intentional odyssey — discovering an alternate route. When "lost" is re-defined this way, neither my direction-giver nor I feel stupid — an important concept in the continuous cognitive-rehab program known as rewiring life.

Attention and concentration. These frequent problem areas are not easily seen in testing or other structured settings. Playing a definite role in these deficit areas is our inability to filter out extraneous or background noise/stimuli. Survivors may be criticized for lack of attention when in fact we're exhausted from trying to screen out distracting noises that others filter out automatically! This may partly explain your survivor's problems with crowds. Survivors seem to have an increased sensitivity to noise, so that all noises seem louder and more invasive than to non-injured others. Ideas on how to deal with intrusive noise can be found in many sections of this book, especially Chapter 4.

Information processing, storage, and retrieval. Survivors may be slow to hear and respond to information. There are also difficulties in storing and retrieving — remembering and finding — information.

Language deficits. Problems with language are common. These include an inability or slowness to understand (*aphasia*), read (*dyslexia*), find words (*anomia*), speak (*dysnomia*), or write the desired word (*dysgraphia*). Stuttering and stammering may also occur at especially stressful times.

What are some executive function areas that are affected?
- Problem solving.
- Judgment.
- Concept formation.
- Mental flexibility.
- Ability to generalize new information and to learn from an experience.
- Ability to understand abstract concepts.
- Assessment of his strengths and weaknesses — possibly the most disabling aspect is that your survivor may be unaware of what is wrong.

With all these deficit areas, can survivors get better?

Yes! Cognitive rehabilitation not only improves thinking ability, but also leads to significant overall improvement. Studies suggest that how well intellectual and memory functions return affects survivors'

> In the middle of difficulty lies opportunity.
> — Albert Einstein

ultimate outcome: return to productive activity and successful reentry to the community — and perhaps even the work force. Most certainly, when survivors increase their cognitive skills, they are better able to emotionally adjust to — maybe even accept — their injuries, in part because they're less disabled! Improvement can't come without a big "if" — "if" brain-injury survivors try!

How long will survivors keep improving?

As long as they work at it — the "use it or lose it" adage is especially appropriate. Even after several years, improvement in all areas has been observed by professionals, loved ones, and survivors (Najenson et al., 1974). And as cognitive

> Words don't move mountains. Work, exacting work, moves mountains.
> — Danilo Dolci

functioning improves, so does emotional and behavioral functioning.

Good news! Recent studies refute earlier theories that most recovery after head injury occurs within the first six months and nearly all of it within the first two years after the injury. In fact, according to more recent research, survivors show continuous improvement in both neurological and functional measures 10-12 years post-injury — including all aspects of function in life: cognitive, motor, social, emotional, and behavioral (Sbordone, 1991). Anecdotal reports are even more impressive: my friend's 80-year-old father who sustained a brain injury over 40 years ago is still doing new things!

Personal experience. *Even after all these years, I continue to improve and often ponder: "How good can I get?" Some people don't know when to quit!*

How can survivors compensate for executive function deficits?
My wise counselor Dr. Christine Baser and I created the SAFER acronym: Stop, Assess, Fix, Examine, Retry. Visualize SAFER on a STOP sign! Before we cross a street, whether the "street" is speaking or acting, first we need to stop what we're doing to assess the situation and develop a plan. Then, we implement the plan to fix it. To determine if it works, we examine/test our plan. If our plan doesn't work, we go back to the beginning to try another plan. If the new plan works, we proceed; if not, we stop again and develop another plan. We repeat this until we develop a strategy that works — or we stop and try again another day. We're not quitting; we're regrouping!

What are the ways to predict degree of recovery?
While predictors of recovery typically include pre-injury personality, degree of neurological damage, and current behavior and environment, current research suggests that the environment — mental, physical, and social stimulation — enhances growth — and therefore recovery!

What are the behavioral and environmental predictors of recovery?
Regardless of a survivor's neurological injuries, certain behaviors can predict recovery: motivation/goal orientation, persistence, independence, concern for others, optimism, and activity. If your survivor exhibits only some of these qualities, focus on those and model/encourage the others.

Success-producing environmental factors include structure, routine, harmony, and repetition in daily activities. Create these vital components at home and seek them in your community by encouraging your survivor to participate in regularly scheduled classes, activities, and services.

What kinds of interactions are most helpful?
As in any learning environment, people who are warm, involved, and supportive reinforce a survivor's motivation and self-esteem, as does an uncritical acceptance of deficits and an unwavering belief that improvement can occur. At those times when you don't feel so accepting and strong, fake it — your survivor probably won't know! It also helps if there is a non-family key person to act as advocate.

Why does cognitive functioning vary so greatly?
It's about that connection between cognitive and emotional functioning!
Conditional neurological lesion is a useful term that describes the
phenomenon — that a survivor's current stress level determines both
cognitive and behavioral responses to any demand (Najenson et al.,
1974). In other words, stress makes us stupid!

Variable conditions from both the past injury and the present
environment likely create these unpredictable responses. Injury factors
include the survivor's age and the nature and extent of the damage.
Current causes involve the amount of emotional stress in whatever calls
for memory as well as fatigue and other metabolic demands, including
amount and timing of food, medication, exercise, and sleep.

*Personal experience. My cognitive abilities, general health, and thus
my emotional state, vary markedly from winter to summer, for a variety
of reasons, including Seasonal Affective Disorder (SAD). When I listen
more to my body and don't push it to run half-marathons or do other
activities that stress me beyond my winter limits, body and brain are
healthier. It only took me twenty-five years to discover this!*

What results from a misunderstood cognitive functioning level?
A variable level of abilities creates frustration, discouragement, and
problems with community reentry — both vocationally and socially. An
inaccurate or incomplete assessment can also lead to inappropriate
decisions by your survivor and by others on his behalf, resulting in
improper placements and unrealistic vocational and financial dreams and
plans.

Which professionals help with cognitive rehabilitation?
Cognitive rehabilitation professionals
include neuropsychologists, occupational
therapists, and speech-language
pathologists. Other therapists may use
cognitive skills in their work. If individual

> I was taught that the
> way of progress is
> neither swift nor easy
> — Marie Curie

or group cognitive therapy is not possible, consult your rehab team or
brain injury foundation for their suggestions about other suitable training.

All these professionals know what to do and how to do it! They use methods that both rely on survivors' strengths and acknowledge their weaknesses — they don't do what doesn't work. They teach strategies to "do what you can with what you have." Special aids/devices that can be used at home are incorporated into cognitive rehabilitation.

Personal experience. *Finally — someone to work with me to fix my brain! In 1988 — 12 years post-injury — as part of the plan to return me to productive employment, Deborah Abrams, PhD, a former Sharp Hospital Work-reentry Coordinator, referred me to the Speech Pathology Department. I worked with Eugenia Don, who was the second professional, after my dear psychologist DJ, to really believe me when I said, "Fix my brain and I won't be crazy."*

Eugenia learned that part of the discrepancy between my perform-ance and test results came about because I was able to respond in a structured environment but not in a time-pressured and non-structured one. So she selected user-friendly yet challenging activities that increased my mental flexibility.

Eugenia and I began our sessions with me unloading the latest emotional problem, her offering either her ear or suggestions or both, and then our getting to work. It is well known that general psychological effects — including reduction of anxiety and frustration — are most important in speech therapy.

We met twice a week for about nine months. Then Eugenia compiled two notebooks with activities that my best friend Marlys and I could do as we drove

> Mind moves matter.
> — Virgil

from California to Minnesota that summer. Even though her calculus-teacher brain already was facile, such brainteasers as "What does the sun do?" and "What are different uses for a paper clip?" engaged both of us. Because Marlys is a math teacher and I always had a good head for math, we saved the math for those times when we needed a lift and could guarantee success. Enjoying our work for up to six hours a day was fun — and my skills improved!

What are cognitive therapy goals and how are they achieved?
Because injury disorganizes the brain and damages thinking abilities, this therapy is designed to both reduce disability and broaden ability to handle information and act on it in a purposeful way. Typically, to rewire and reorganize the brain, survivors learn to:
- Strengthen their remaining abilities.
- Rebuild and relearn basic skills.
- Develop new strategies to compensate for lost skills.

What does research say about cognitive rehabilitation?
Many studies over the years have demonstrated that cognitive rehabilitation leads to improved thinking, which results in better functioning in all areas of life. Because the brain is the control center for the whole body, improvement in cognitive functioning leads to involvement and improvement in all other types of treatment. Working with trained therapists to help survivors improve their mental functioning is a key factor to their successful climb up the rehab mountain.

What are other helpful cognitive connections?
It depends if your survivor prefers people or machines. In addition to cognitive rehabilitation training with rehab professionals, some skilled practitioners use neurofeedback training to harmonize brain wave patterns. Other options include computer programs that offer a variety of levels, structure, immediate feedback, and make learning fun.

Community colleges may also offer classes specifically for brain injury survivors. Even if there is no designated class, general remedial classes also work on skill deficits.

Suggestions for making cognitive connections at home.
Work at home? Yes! It is not only a productive use of time, but also reinforces learning from therapy sessions, which speeds up the recovery process. It may take a lot of experimenting, but I guarantee that something will work! Know that patience and faith are vital, regardless of which methods are used — patience for the long journey and faith that it will get better. Rewiring can happen — if we all work at it.

If your survivor says, "But "I'll be 30 (or 40 or 50) before I... (learn that, finish that degree, etc.),"" respond with "How old will you be if you don't?"

Strategies to improve survivor's cognitive functioning.
- List contents on the front of all cupboards, drawers, and closets. Shorten the lists as memory improves — a visible sign of success!
- Make to-do lists with step-by-step plans.
- Divide large mental or physical tasks into a series of smaller ones. Small steps lead to success!
- Talk, do, then review. Discuss written plans, do tasks together, assess. Use the SAFER method. At another time, observe your survivor while he follows directions and assist him with them.
- Remind your survivor to employ all senses to reinforce memory.
- Design short and easy projects with a measurable end product.
- Reaffirm the team concept, using words like "What if we do..." or "Let's do...."
- Do word and/or number games together.
- Use and encourage positive self-talk "Good!" "That's it!" "You're getting it!"

Hint: If projects are too long or involved, frustration and quitting can result — regardless of how smart your survivor is. Use the word "work" to eliminate emotional overload — "Will that work?"

Personal experience. *Friends can serve as a live thesaurus — it's not a dinosaur! My closest friend and adopted sister, Marlys Henke, used an effective technique every time we talked, either in person or on the phone. When I'd get stuck and needed to search for the correct word, I'd say, "It's an "S" word" — or whatever letter the word started with. She would search her brain's thesaurus for "S" words — and eventually we'd find the right one. We rejoiced because we both felt a sense of accomplishment — and I began to recapture my previous high-level vocabulary. Many people may not enjoy this search-and-find game — but special people do!*

Hint: It's a big help if someone says, "Do you mean ...or...or...?" If words are listed one at a time, they can be either accepted or rejected. It may even become a game for friends to try to guess what word is intended. Your survivor can feel good too as he locates buried vocabulary words and once again can communicate accurately.

What are the basic steps to learn a skill?
- The learner receives instruction in the specific skill.
- The instructor models/demonstrates the skill.
- The learner practices the skill with or without assistance.
- The instructor offers feedback.
- The learner continues to practice the skill, revising if necessary.

Environmental Factors

To help with cognitive rewiring we start with the environment because brains, like flowers, need air, water, light, and nutrients to bloom — plus appropriate music! To ensure a successful work-at-home setting, our focus is two-fold: to reduce the disability and broaden the ability. Examine both internal (food, vitamins, medications, sleep, exercise) and external factors.

Because survivors are not able to screen out incidental sounds, to reduce disability, special learner-friendly music or white noise ensures a successful environment. Notice the difference in your survivor when appropriate music is played. Other distracting noises from any

> The power of music to integrate and cure... is quite fundamental. [It is the] profoundest non-chemical medication.
> — Oliver Sachs

source — especially talking — need to be eliminated during work hours and even when we communicate with others. To recover from the overload of life, survivors need more rest and sleep than non-disabled others.

Suggestions for learning success:
- Keep the environment quiet, well-lighted, and peaceful. Provide structure, routine, frequent breaks, and a slow or unhurried pace.

- Play special music or use white noise (like a fan) to block out distracting bursts of noise.
- Choose the best time of day. Mornings — when people are fresh — are usually best, but not too early — sometime after 9 AM.
- Pace and structure activities to include rest/quiet periods during the day. Alternate more active and less-active days, if needed.
- Be sure your survivor is rested, relaxed, and receptive. Remember that survivors tend to overload easily (too much information, choices, noise, people, activity, etc.) and tend to fade/fatigue in the early evening.
- Be a receptive teacher — be willing to practice and offer feedback in other real life settings. Adjust choices as needs change. Project optimism, continue to seek humor, and remember that sun follows rain — even when the rain seems endless!

Noise-filtering devices:
- Music or white noise
- Headphones with soothing music or just as a filter.
- Ask audiologists/doctors about customized reverse-hearing aids.
- Generic ear plugs.

Prosthetic Memory Devices and External Aids

Artificial intelligence for survivors of brain injury? Why not? We need it more than anyone! Everyone else uses a variety of external brain boosters — from day planners to computers and cell phones — in their daily lives. Computer programs called *cognitive orthotic devices* are

> Results! Why, man, I have gotten a lot of results! I know several thousand things that won't work.
> — Thomas Edison

especially useful to provide a structure for work tasks (Parente, 1991). See Chapter 12 for details. Electronic brains to the rescue!

Kinds of prosthetic memory aids. Check your local electronic and computer stores. See Resources for lists of vendors.

Electronic aids include:
- Signaling devices to help locate keys, wallets, purses, or cars.
- Devices to store personal information and signal appointments.

- Personal directories to store message alarms/reminders.
- Microcassette recorders — manual or voice-activated.

Cognitive training tools/computer applications.
Many tools to improve your survivor's cognitive functioning await your exploration! While therapy notebooks and textbooks provide reliable rehabilitation, computer programs and games add variety.

Various software programs not only offer relevant and functional repetitive skill-building work that demands attention, but they also provide that crucial sense of control — all in an impassive interactive medium. Sometimes it's easier for survivors to deal with predictable and emotionally undemanding machines than with people, even though computers only accept exact responses — which can be very frustrating! Another valuable side-benefit is that computers don't mind verbal abuse! (Levin, 1991).

Various computer approaches include:
- Computer-assisted cognitive rehabilitation (CACR) is invaluable to relearn general skills and to acquire new specific skills.
- Computer games are a fun way to improve cognitive skills, like the Happy Neuron game program, which stimulates attention, memory, and visual-spatial and executive-function skills.
- Shell-system orthotic devices are specialized computer programs that simplify complex tasks and manage daily tasks.
- Simulations provide practice in real-life situations in a protective entertaining environment, like some specialized video games. They can help to both demonstrate and measure learner skills.
- Drill and practice — specific and simple tasks that require repetition — help to relearn buried information. Many choices are available that include skill drills for language, arithmetic, reaction time, attention, reasoning, and visual-spatial abilities.

What does research say about computer use in rehab?
Let's use whatever tools may help! Several studies showed that participants prefer computers for instruction, survivors who received computer memory training showed significant and lasting gains, and people who previously had demonstrated visual-spatial neglect were able

to improve their reading, attention, and other visual-spatial abilities. Significantly, studies showed that those who were most impaired improved to the level of those least impaired on computerized cognitive training tasks! (Levin, 1991).

Computer-environment set-up.
- Create an ergonomic, pleasing, and well-lit workspace.
- Track balls offer many benefits over regular mice.
- Experiment with different kinds and heights of keyboards.
- Invest in a large screen to improve display.
- Contact local and on-line stores for a variety of programs.
- Voice-recognition software can be helpful for people with visual-spatial and/or hand-coordination problems.

Table Games

Play a game — what an enjoyable way to learn or practice a skill! Modifying some rules — forming teams — can ensure both fun and success. Although specific skills needed may vary, all games require attention, perception, sequencing, memory, and problem solving.

Perhaps the most important benefits of games are that the repetition is enjoyable — it doesn't seem like work, social interaction is required, and games are played by non-injured folks — so are not considered to be "therapy." Games are also fun, inexpensive, available, adaptable, rewarding, meaningful, familiar to many people, variable, non-threatening, and available with adjustable difficulty levels. Specific skills and the games that emphasize them (Deaton, 1991) include:
- Attention: Bingo and card games such as Slapjack, Uno, Crazy Eights.
- Perceptual skills: Bingo, Checkers, Candyland, Gridlock.
- Sequencing: Boggle, Numbers Up, Poker, Dominoes, Scrabble, Scrabble Sentence Cubes, Numbers Up Simon, solitaire, Sudoku.
- Memory: Concentration, Memory, Enchanted Forest.
- Long-term memory: Whatzit?, Trivial Pursuit, Win-Lose-Draw.
- Problem-solving: Connect Four, Who Dun it?, Clue, Scruples, Scattergories.
- Visual discrimination: Battleship, Boggle, Guess Who?, Jenga.

Other Games

- Specialized video games can be a fun and social way to improve skills.
- Manual games such as Ping Pong, pool, and Foosball all require hand-eye coordination and dexterity. Creative adaptations can level the playing field; for example, the more skillful player can play with his non-dominant hand or be allowed fewer mistakes.
- Life can be a game! Virtually anything, including chores, can be made into a game with rewards. You can vary the time, alternate the tasks, or change the colors or number of turns to create fun out of work!

Friends as Tutors

It takes a special person to be able to tutor a survivor who previously had high skills. Family and pre-injury friends often cannot emotionally disengage themselves from the loss sufficiently to effectively work with the survivor. The nature of the relationship is changed — it is no longer "even." If you are unable to work with

> The vocal nourishment that a mother provides to her child is just as important to the child's development as her milk.
> — Alfred Tomatis, MD

your survivor, find someone who can, such as the children of old friends. They may be more than happy to tutor him — it enables them to be teachers instead of students for a change! They feel good and your survivor enjoys them — it's another win-win situation!

Personal experience. Sadly, I recall my oldest and dearest friend's attempt to mask a pained expression on her face when her daughter and I began to work on a simple therapy task. She excused herself — perhaps horrified to see what her cherished childhood friend had lost. She was kind to me, provided meals, didn't expect much, and always invited me to join with her and her girls in outings. Her strong faith is likely a big reason she didn't abandon me.

But her other friends thought me strange and asked her embarrassing questions — but because of our great love for one another, she continued to be my friend. She still visited me in the various hospitals, even venturing into the locked ward one time — traumatized but there for me. However, it was obvious that I had become a burden instead of a joy.

Communication Do's and Don'ts for Loved ones

Directness is the only way to communicate with many survivors. It takes courage, and probably means returning to less sophisticated ways of talking, but needs to be done.

However, remember that "sticks and stones do break my bones and words can hurt me" — word choice with survivors is as important as with any developing individual. Set him up for success with encouraging words!

- Do ask only one question at a time. This is very difficult for smart people to do, whether survivor or helper — and it is very important!
- Don't ask a question that includes more than one choice. Asking "Do you want to walk at the park or would you rather go to the mall?" short-circuits a survivor's brain because we still need to remember to answer the first question after we've heard the second.
- Do ask specific questions.
- Do encourage the survivor to decide things.
- Don't argue with his choice.
- Do help him analyze his needs for a calendar, pen, bus schedule, notebook, etc.
- Don't question what he tells you. Don't say, "Why do you need that?"
- Do ask questions about his choice — "How have you set yourself up to succeed? What is plan B, in case plan A doesn't work? What is Plan C?" etc.
- Do ask what happened. Help him analyze it and what, if anything, he'll do differently the next time, e.g., write information down in a notebook, leave earlier, etc.
- Don't criticize him or what happened. Don't say, "That was a stupid thing to do."
- Do model appropriate behavior — practice what you preach!
- Don't reinforce child-like behaviors.
- Do reinforce adult behaviors.

- Do remind him to use helpful and kindly self-talk.
- Don't rescue him. Don't remember for him or do something for him.
- For your mental health and his, do spend time away from your survivor.

Do's and Don'ts — Word Choices

- Do say: "I know you'll do your best", "I know you can do it", and "I have confidence in you."
- Don't say: "Why can't you just...", "Why can't you grow up?", or "What's wrong with you?"
- Do say: "You did a good job on...", "You look really nice", or "What do you think about...."

> Before we speak, our words should pass through three gates. Is it true? Is it kind? Is it necessary?
> — Ancient Oriental Wisdom

- Don't say in a critical way: "Why did you do that?" or "Why didn't you...?"
- Do say: "What do you want to say?" or "Another way could be..."
- Don't say: "Why did you say that?"
- Do say: "What bothers you?"
- Don't say: "How can that bother you? It's nothing!"

When you are talking with your survivor use the key words: how, we, need, work, and what/how questions

- The word "how" is an action word and not blame-oriented.
- Using "we" implies a partnership and that no one needs to solve the problem alone.
- The words "need" and "work" remove any emotional overtones to the task. All jobs "need" certain things for success.
- "What" and "how" require your survivor to examine what isn't working and tells you what needs to be changed — the SAFER method.

Examples:

- Ask: "What do we need to do for this to work for you?" or "How can we make this work for you?"

- Check if it's working with a question: "How is this working?"
- If it's not working, ask: "What do we need to change to make it work?", "Will this work?", or "If I do this, will this work?"
- Do not accept "I don't know" as an answer.
- If the question seems too overwhelming, say: "Let's figure out just what part isn't working. Is it…?" Then list the parts, one by one, until he picks one. This will bring success for all!

Summary

- The brain can grow new cells and form new networks.
- One side of the brain can compensate for the other side.
- An interesting environment will spur new growth.
- Survivors keep improving as long as they work at it.
- Improvement in cognitive functioning leads to involvement and improvement in all other types of treatment.
- Make to-do lists with step-by-step plans and review them.
- Design short and easy projects with a measurable end product.
- Work word and number games together.
- Play special learner-friendly music or white noise.
- Play games as an enjoyable way to learn or practice a skill.
- Ask only one question at a time.
- Help him analyze his needs.
- Don't question what he tells you.
- Do ask: **"How have you set yourself up to succeed?"**
- Model appropriate behavior and pay attention to your word choice.
- Use and encourage positive self-talk.

6

Emotional Rewiring: Healing His Feelings and Spirits

It isn't for the moment you are stuck that you need courage, but for the long, uphill climb back to sanity and faith and security.
— Anne Morrow Lindbergh

In one sense, brain injury survivors are like all trauma survivors — they simply want to endure the next minute or hour or day, one breath at a time, and improve their health, one step at a time. Reserves are depleted. Batteries are drained. Exposed nerves scream in terror at the mere thought of contact. Heightened and confused senses simultaneously broadcast and receive. Absolutely nothing and no one can enter their space unless they benefit. Their entire life focus and all energy must go into survival and rehabilitation — or it won't happen. Using an ocean metaphor, in this chapter we discuss:

- Causes of emotional and psychosocial problems.
- Responses to emotional and psychosocial problems.
- Grief and loss: stages of grief and dimensions of loss.
- Substance use and abuse; treatments.
- Self-harm and suicide.
- Helpful/non-helpful behaviors during the grieving process.
- Family rewiring.

Introduction

While similar in some respects, brain-injury survivors and those who experience other types of trauma also have significant differences. Brain injury survivors' deepest wounds are invisible and hidden — at times even from themselves. Subtle though their wounds may be, they linger, changeable from hour to hour and from day to day — like the ocean. But they, the wounded persons, are not like the ocean in its timely tidal flow, unfazed by wind or rain, sun or storm.

Survivors are the tempestuous sea, shaped by seasonal elements. Winter wipes them out like surfers in a tsunami and summer seduces them like swimmers in swells. They're affected by such atmospheric conditions as wind and cloud cover and storms from afar. Their surf can be choppy on the surface and calm near the bottom — if they dive deep enough to power through the turbulence.

There, the ocean floor is strangely tranquil beneath all the turmoil and confusion. The fine-grained sand is soft and inviting — and safe. No demons lurk there. No danger exists. But they cannot linger without oxygen, so they look up at the sun for the signal that the turbulence has passed and the coast is clear. So, refreshed and renewed, they resurface — for now. They know that they can return to the calm whenever their wounds need flushing, whenever they cry out in pain — or just whenever they choose. Survivors are often like the sea that is smooth as glass in the morning and in the evening — before and after the daily turbulence.

Although survivors' wounds and pain tolerance may vary, what doesn't change is their overall health and sanity — it remains elusive. They may look fine, but they're not fine — not quite. So they can't act fine all the time. Survivors rejoice in their fine moments; for some of them those moments become hours, days — even weeks occasionally, when they're on a real good run. At these times, their disability is almost forgotten. They seduce others, and even themselves, into the belief that they've achieved a balanced lifestyle and are happy with where they are.

Then, all aglow with success, they review their status and suddenly realize — something important is missing! It's work or school one time; play another. It could be love, absent so long it's easily forgotten. So, full of confidence and unaccustomed ease, they seek that one last part of the puzzle. But it's too far away.

Their attempts to reach a higher level empty not only their ready fuel but their storage tanks as well. Adrenaline-loaded, they don't even feel the subtle signs of impending doom — let alone know to heed them! Sickness descends with a storm-like fury. They need to shut down and rest, go back to the basics. But they want more! They saw how wonderful life can be with everything in perfect balance — and they liked it. They want to return to that.

Damned disability — it didn't want to be forgotten! It stayed hidden just long enough to deceive even them. Balance was touched and even hugged — but vaporized before it securely connected — this time!

What happened? They didn't maintain perfect balance — despite their best attempts to camouflage their flaws and others' efforts to ignore them — because they're still damaged. Nothing can change that, at least not yet. Maybe one day someone will create super brain-glue to heal all wounds.

While you seek that glue, perhaps the best hope at this time is to find an angel or two who knows your survivor is wounded and likes him anyway. Together, you can repair some broken areas and conceal others to display his best side. Eventually, perhaps, the damage will fade in importance, if not in appearance, to everyone.

That injury occurred must be believed or the health that is elusive becomes either lost or destroyed. Perhaps it boils down to this: *I cannot spend my life trying to convince people something is — or isn't — wrong and still have enough time and energy to fix it!*

Personal experience. *In the 1970s, before MRIs, if damage couldn't be seen on an X-ray, it didn't exist. So, even with abnormal EEG readings and despite a repeatedly measured 30-point spread between my verbal and performance IQ, my moderate-and-diffuse brain injury did not exist! That I had been a teacher and coach was not considered. I knew something was wrong with my brain but, because it was thought that I hadn't recovered from a recent divorce, I was labeled emotionally labile and histrionic — the medical profession's explanation for my behavior in the sexist 1970s! That my face and body was black-and-blue* *from head to toe was not considered important — I was simply nuts, bouncing from one psych ward to another, always heavily sedated so I wouldn't decompensate and explode!*

So, Carolyn-the-coach tried to get physical help — surely they can see I need help with my weak right side — later tested at 30% weaker than my left!. I assumed wrong! I remember one night in the psych ward when I demanded an immediate neurological exam because my arm collapsed as I attempted a pushup. After the doctor's quick exam — "touch your nose with your finger and grasp my thumb" (real tough for an athlete!) the unforgettable words: "Nothing is the matter." I probably needed heavy sedation that night!

As a result of the nothing's-wrong diagnosis, the medical response when I requested physical therapy was to display stroke survivors who struggled to walk up the ramp. Then I heard "you're not bad enough" because I could walk to rehab. Apparently no one noticed the wide gait I'd developed so that I could walk without falling, my clumsiness, or my postural imbalances. Never mind that my weak side was never tested again, despite my histrionics.

I looked fine but wasn't fine — and no one would believe me. I truly was going nuts, hastened by medical professionals who simply wouldn't believe something was wrong without tangible scientific evidence. The fact that my behavior offered very strong proof apparently was not enough — until I met Dale Johnson, PhD, a psychologist at the Texas Tech Psychosomatic Clinic in El Paso. (How I landed in Texas on my way from Minnesota to California is another story.)

One of my first angels, Dr. Johnson believed me — and saved my life. I called him "DJ" because I didn't like doctors and I wanted to like him. He was my last hope. DJ believed I would thrive and rattled my cage so that I would survive. I honored his faith in me by "knocking on doors ... as many as it takes" and never, ever giving up on me or anybody else. Sadly, I lost DJ — damn cigarettes — to "the Big C" in 1990.

Can anything be learned from this story? Hopefully, professionals are now more aware that a lack of positive test results may simply reflect neurodiagnostic tests' lack of sensitivity and/or specificity for what is measured. In other words, it's the fault of the tests, and not the testee!

The adage "absence of proof is not proof of absence" is very appropriate here! (Zasler, 1992).

My saga also illustrates why the "long, uphill climb back to sanity and faith and security" is so difficult. The visible and invisible backpacks that survivors carry, filled with the residue of injury, are exceptionally heavy.

It is no surprise, then, that emotional and behavioral problems can become the most significant and lasting effect of brain injury (Prigatano, 1995; Hendryx, 1989) — and by far the most limiting effect on social and community re-integration. Let's explore what research tells us about this most challenging aspect — and what you can do about it.

Emotional/Psychosocial Problems

Causes

You learned about the chemical soup that surrounds the brain in Chapter 3. You can understand why even those with the mildest trauma often exhibit inappropriate behavior once this balance is disturbed.

Many of these behaviors result from physical brain damage, both the direct and the secondary effects — they are not intentional or the fault of the survivor. Likewise, symptoms cannot be classified into either a physical or a psychiatric cause.

Scientists disagree about the sources of the maladaptive behavior. Some researchers look to the injury of the frontal lobe (e.g., Prigatano, 1995). Others suggest that temporal lobe injuries are more likely to produce psychiatric disability (Sbordone, 1991). Still others connect behavioral problems to left hemisphere injuries.

Experts agree, however, that a wide range of emotional and psychosocial problems are not related to either the location or the severity of the injury. It is now recognized that many aberrant behaviors — agitation, aggression, perseveration, apathy, distractibility — reflect the underlying cognitive impairment that results from the organic damage. For example, altered attention can produce confusion and impaired memory, which can lead to agitation.

Responses

How someone behaves after a neurological insult like a brain injury is a function of the degree to which that person is under stress, fatigue, emotional distress, or excessive metabolic demands from their trauma (Sbordone, 1987). This conclusion reminds us again of the importance of a peaceful environment.

Four typical kinds of emotional responses have been identified: loss of self-esteem and self-confidence, denial, anxiety, and depression. Others include irritability, moodiness, apathy, increased sensitivity to stress, isolation, inflexibility, paranoia/delusions, and poor interaction skills.

In response to their feelings, survivors may exhibit these behaviors: aggression, agitation, restlessness, distractibility, temper outbursts, compulsions, impulsivity, frustration, sexual acting-out, childish behaviors, and egocentricity. *Whew — what a list, huh?*

Interestingly, these same behaviors are often exhibited in response to the death of a loved one. Trauma reactions can be like grief responses. So, your survivor is not nuts — he's grieving — a big difference! What often occurs is a behavior change — often a regression — of the whole personality with pre-injury temperament and traits more pronounced after the injury. In other words, if he was assertive, he might become aggressive; and if he was shy, he might become reclusive.

Studies also show that a survivor's behavior may take one of two opposite directions: focusing frustration outward (outbursts, irritability, and lack of impulse control) or inward (apathy, isolation, and depression), depending on the neurological damage. See also Chapter 11.

One of the most challenging aspects of dealing with survivors is quick mood swings — *aren't you lucky!* Because of the variety of ways someone can be injured, it is difficult to predict which deficits he may exhibit, or when, or if, or how. Different injuries lead to different states.

Finally, to further confuse everyone, which problem behavior occurs and how extreme the behavior is can vary throughout the day as well as from day to day!

Can survivors improve?

Yes — there is hope! After learning about all the problems, a common response is, "Okay. I know it's bad. But is there any hope? Will he get better?"

Yes — not like he was, but better — and everyone plays an important role in that recovery. Let's repair the loose screws that cause the attention deficit rather than sentence survivors to the psych ward or a lifetime on anti-psychotics! *"Just fix my brain and I won't be crazy!"*

Don't blame him! Please realize and believe that he's doing the best he can! If he could act more appropriately, he would. Most survivors don't want to be crazy — after the initial "ain't it awful" period, there is little worthwhile payback for acting strangely. Typically, bad behavior is first tolerated by others, and then avoided. So, let's correct behavior that's ineffective. Then he can move from being tolerated to being accepted.

Knowledge of research helps us to see with scientists' eyes, to see that a behavior is at fault — not the person. Undesirable behaviors do not need to be accepted, Survivors can be trained if we know what to do. We can look objectively at the problem as something to be fixed rather than somebody to be fixed — using the necessary steps in between. For example, say, "Instead of [what he's doing], what I want is [the desired action]." Then say, "Good. That's closer. You're getting it."

His environment can either help or hinder him. Evidence shows that the emotional and motivational states of survivors often determine the extent and rate of their recovery.

Keys for improvement.

Rebuilding self-esteem at this stage of life is similar to developing it in his first few years of life. He needs:

- Rewarding interactions with others through which his needs are met.
- A feeling of mastery over his world through his accomplishments and skills, from which he develops future plans.

Courage is not innate — it develops step by step. Help rebuild his confidence in mastering small tasks, then courage to master big ones naturally follows.

Grief and Loss

The Stages of Grief

For a full discussion, see *Brain Injury Rewiring for Survivors.*

The first stage: denial.
Although generally accepted as the first stage in the grief process, denial may occur anytime, may be brief, or may never occur at all. If he frequently used denial to cope with life before injury, then it is likely he will rely on it to cope with life now.

   What to do: Because a feeling of hope is necessary for any degree of recovery, it is vital to use words that neither dash hope nor affirm and reward denial. Your survivor is testing everyone and everything in his environment to see what and whom he can trust, so truthfulness is crucial. For him to remain in denial for an extended period will not help him. Validating statements that are untrue can prolong this stage. Denial is usually a temporary wayside on the road to acceptance. While feeling hopeful is necessary for any degree of recovery, it is unhealthy to remain in denial for an extended period.

The second stage: anger.
To understand the source of the anger, simply put yourself in his shoes. What if all your plans, hopes, and dreams were suddenly thwarted, and replaced with the struggle to talk or think or move? What if you were lying in bed, unable to move, with tubes everywhere, watching people hustle in and out of your room? And, so you're not accused of being difficult, you submit to yet another test to demonstrate that something else is wrong. No wonder he's angry with everyone and everything!

   What to do: While it is easy to be defensive, react negatively, and attack his frequent angry outbursts, your behavior just reaffirms his belief that he's unlovable and nobody cares. Attempt to understand the source of his fury, respect his need to be angry, and don't respond personally to it. Suggest anger-defusing activities such as those described later in this chapter.

Again, use our SAFER method: Stop. Assess — determine the trigger for the anger. Fix — brainstorm how to alter or avoid that circumstance and setting in the future. Examine the effectiveness of your plan. Retry new alternatives and repeat the SAFER process if necessary.

For personal safety, protect yourself from physical harm. Seek the help of a mental-health professional when your survivor demonstrates any of the following behaviors (Baser, 1997):

- Suicidal threats/attempts — even joking.
- Substance abuse.
- Aggressive behavior or verbal threats.
- Compulsive behaviors — rituals or repeated actions without cause, like hand washing or checking on an item, that interfere with daily activities.
- Refusal to attend therapy, take essential medication, or follow a previously agreed upon care plan or medical instructions.

The third stage: bargaining.

While false hope is not beneficial, survivors in this stage are highly motivated, enthusiastic about therapy, and willing to work.

What to do: Help him to remain hopeful that progress is possible by encouraging continued hard work. For example, rather than saying, "If you do this, you'll be able to…", say, "If you do this, you'll have a better chance at…" Also, saying "If you don't do this, you probably won't be able to…" can be used occasionally if it motivates your survivor. However, unrealistic expectations can result in him getting stuck at this stage — which delays learning compensatory strategies and self-acceptance.

The fourth stage: depression.

By this stage, all the previous behaviors are replaced by a sense of great loss and hopelessness. This is a normal and natural reaction, not just to a stressful and traumatic event but also to the devastation of the injury.

Kinds of depression.

Reactive or situational depression. Your survivor may display behaviors like those who experience a severe disappointment such as job loss, financial reversal, divorce. Usual responses run the gamut from withdrawal and need for space to a need for verbal interaction and sharing. There may be a strong need to express feelings — by outward means such as talking, crying, screaming, hitting, etc.

What to do: Optimism and attempts to cheer, encourage, or reassure usually help with this kind of depression. "Yes, you're still lovable." "It wasn't your fault," etc. However, excessive cheerfulness can make things worse.

Clinical depression may be identified by both depth and duration of response. As you see in the following list, some symptoms are polar opposites (like major weight loss versus weight gain). Note, too, that clinical depression varies from situational depression not just in the number of symptoms but also the length of time they are present.

What to do: Confer with a neuropsychologist if you wonder whether a reaction is beyond what might be expected in terms of both depth and duration of response. Trust your instincts. It is very important that clinical depression is treated and not allowed to worsen. Don't make the mistake of "just give him time and he'll get over it." Time may cause further deterioration and can lead to self-destructive behaviors. While there are many causes of depression, there may be a chemical imbalance that medication could correct.

Seek professional help if he demonstrates at least five of the following behaviors for two weeks (Taber, 1989):

- Near-total loss of interest in most areas of life that previously brought pleasure, such as food, sex, work, friends, hobbies, or entertainment.
- Poor appetite and significant weight loss or major weight gain.
- Motoric slowing or agitation.
- No need or excessive need for sleep.
- Lack of energy or fatigue.
- Problems with concentration.
- Feelings of worthlessness or excessive guilt.
- Expressed thoughts of death or suicide. — Get immediate help if he talks about attempting or actually attempts suicide!
- Withdrawal.

Preparatory depression mourns future and impending losses and is more of a deep sadness. Although this type of depression is more typical of — and necessary for — those who are terminally ill to reach some state of final acceptance, a brain-injury survivor — and the survivor's loved ones too — may need this time for reflection.

What to do: Helpful expressions of condolence include a touch, a hug, or just silent companionship — there may be little need for words. Preparatory depression is different in nature from situational depression and needs to be dealt with differently. It does not benefit from encouragement and reassurance. In

> Before we speak, our words should pass through three gates: Is it true? Is it kind? Is it necessary?
> — ancient Oriental Proverb

fact, well-meaning folks can interfere with a survivor's emotional preparation if they constantly tell him not to be sad. Your survivor may say something like "It is a very sad thing that happened, and I'm afraid that …" "Don't tell me not to be sad or not to worry!"

The fifth stage: acceptance

In this stage, there are neither good nor bad feelings, but an understanding of the outcome, if not the implications, of the loss.

Acceptance does not necessarily mean accepting limitations — it only means accepting the situation. Gone forever are hoping for a better recovery, trying every rehab center in the country, and waiting for a new drug, surgery, neurological

> To be what we are, and to become what we are capable of becoming, is the only end of life.
> — Baruch Spinoza

discovery, or spending every minute on research or every dollar on the latest "brain fix." Gone are denying and bargaining. Even anger and depression find a new outlet. Grieving isn't over — it's just focused in a new direction. No more waiting! It's time for acting, for experimenting, for trying new things.

At this stage, survivors are often very motivated and actively strive for improvement. Focus and energy are directed toward rehabilitation. Recovery work centers on strengthening some abilities, compensating for deficits, and adapting the environment.

What to do: If your survivor acknowledges even a small degree of acceptance of limitations — "Okay, if this is what I have to work with, how can I make it work better?" — introduce him to devices and techniques that are designed to improve functioning.

Personal experience. Even a sem-blance of acceptance allows me to listen when reality speaks. As my beloved neuropsychologist, Christine Baser, PhD,

> The only failure is not to try.
> — Patricia Weir

gently reminded me, I still have limitations — not every wall can be climbed over, burrowed under, scurried around, or bullied through. I am, after all, still somewhat disabled — although I hate to admit it. I am okay — I'm just different from what I was. That doesn't stop me from trying — relentlessly! — to be the best that I can be.

Dimensions of Loss

Brain injury results in many different kinds of losses. As you and your survivor travel — and get stuck — in the grief cycle, you will find differences in your responses to these losses.

There are five distinct types of loss: loss of significant person/other, loss of external object, developmental loss, loss of security, and loss of some aspect of self (Tanner, 1984). See *Brain Injury Rewiring for Survivors* for a more thorough discussion of loss.

Loss of significant person/valued other. Your survivor is not who he was. The one you knew is missing — not only from his own life, but also from the lives of family and friends — as if he were dead. While he is not actually gone, his decreased ability to communicate causes a psychological separation — handicapping connections between him and everyone in his life. This psychological separation may be more keenly felt than actual physical separation because the survivor is

> I had lost my best friend, my lover, my husband, and the father of my children, but because he was physically present, that loss was not readily recognized by anyone. I missed the friendship, intimacy, and sexual fulfillment that our marriage had held.
> — Marty Beaver

physically present — which serves as a reminder both of what was and what is now. Without mutual problem solving, everyone experiences a profound sense of loss.

Loss of external object and/or abilities affects your survivor and his loved ones.
This aspect of loss may not be felt immediately. It is value-based — the greater the treasure, the greater the loss. Not just the object is missed — part of the value is symbolic. The grief reaction that a missing object evokes can remind someone that he has lost abilities associated with that object. For example, when a survivor is removed from his home and placed in a hospital or nursing home, the result is often homesickness for his entire environment and everything it represents.

Personal experience. In my pre-injury life, I loved to sew and do crafts. I remember crying inside when my mother's best friend arrived at the hospital with a craft kit because it required fine motor coordination that I no longer possessed. Later, it saddened me to see it around, so I gave it away. As is typical, for years I denied my diminished abilities. About ten years after my injury I even purchased a sewing machine, thinking enough time had passed, thinking: "Surely, I can sew now!" Ten years later, it had never been used — my despair included a wasted $300 and anger at a false assumption!

Developmental loss.
This loss, normally associated with the aging process, seems to be the least important, though tremendous grief is felt by survivors because of the "instant aging" caused by the injury. Gone are hopes of being the next singing sensation or professional athlete. Although both young and old experience this type of loss, the loss is actually felt more in older persons, who become more aware of the accelerated aging process.

Loss of security.
Life's predictability was replaced by anxiety over uncontrollable factors. Both you and your survivor feel powerless. Once confident and secure, now he is anxious and doesn't know what to do — or even what could be done. Lack of security is a direct result both of the brain injury and the

accompanying changes in lifestyle, residence, and control. Uncertainty over present and future financial well-being affects the whole family.

Loss of some aspect of self.
Wide in scope and significance, this includes diminished and/or lost intellectual, emotional, and physical functions. Prominent changes may have occurred: executive-function deficits, sensory dysfunctions, paralysis or weakness of one or both sides of the body, chronic pain, emotional instability (increased irritability, apathy, and anxiety) lost or diminished sense of self-worth, change in sex drive, and deficits in the ability to communicate, remember, learn, and concentrate.

Loved Ones and Grieving

It's the typical grief scene. First, shock, then denial, followed by worry and confusion — often all at the same time.

"Oh no! My poor....Who is this person? This is not my loved one! Will he be all right? What can I do? What's going to happen?"

No kidding! — Your survivor isn't alone in his grief. You all feel the loss of your former relationships and lifestyle, your past hopes and dreams. While each loved one feels the loss separately, grieves differently, and needs to mourn — alone — in his or her own way, the family as a unit needs to mourn — together — for what was lost. See *Brain Injury Rewiring for Survivors* Chapter 6 for various healing rituals to inspire you to create your own memorial rites.

After the shared grieving experience, keep the lines of communication open. Talk about how to incorporate the former hopes, dreams, and goals into a revised plan for "the new person with the same name."

Do not ignore or deny the loss — embrace it, for you too need to give yourselves permission to grieve. Seek ways to feel sorrow and to find meaning — only then can you and your loved ones regain a sense of order, control, and purpose as you all reconstruct your lives. Only then can the loss be integrated into the revised life version. Therapy can also help as discussed below.

Loved ones' responses affect your survivor.

As flowers either flourish or perish, depending on their hardiness and the soil where they're planted, survivors rely on their earth — their home environment — to thrive. When flowers receive too much or too little water and fertilizer, they

> Grief can't be worked out if people don't talk about the person who has died.
> — William Pinsof

suffer. So it is with your survivor — your responses can nurture, drown, or starve the vulnerable seedling.

As natural as it is, communicating your feelings of shock, guilt, denial, confusion, depression, resentment, and rejection slows the healing process. It's best to do your grieving without putting the burden of it on your survivor. Remember that showing warmth, faith, acceptance, and resilience positively affects recovery.

Psychological benefits of grieving.

Stop the clocks, turn all mirrors to the walls, cease all work, bring out the clay pipes and whiskey — it's time to mourn the death of our beloved.

While some people consider mourning rites outmoded or unnecessary in today's fast-paced era, such rituals can aid the grieving process. Acknowledgment moves us out of the denial mode.

Beliefs about the healing benefits of grieving have changed over the years — from severing ties to keeping them. Psychologists now realize that breaking all connections to someone or something deeply loved is not natural or healthy — if keeping the bond doesn't hinder the griever from seeking new attachments and interests. In fact, remembering a beloved departed one may provide courage, motivate someone to keep a promise, or inspire someone to achieve a goal.

Helpful and unhelpful behaviors during the grieving process.

Grieving is very painful, as people who have lost something or someone dear can attest. Survivors may have no prior experience of loss or of dependency caused by injury. Thus, when the devastating impact of a brain injury occurs, they may not know how to cope. It is my hope that the following suggestions, painfully learned, will help your journey.

What Not To Do

Offering false cheer. Attempts to cheer your survivor — and yourself — by saying, "Well, it could be worse. You could have died. Look at what you have left. What are you complaining about?" could result in him talking less, bottling up more, and becoming even more depressed.

Reframing the problem as yours. "How do you think I like it? Now all my time is spent caring for you!" Do not add the burden of how hard it is for you on top of his own struggle.

Denying. Continued attempts to distract him are not helpful at the depression stage, however beneficial they were earlier.

Avoiding. Not dealing with the changes does not bring anyone closer to getting on with life. Be honest and walk the talk.

Enabling. Initially, showing sympathy with the "poor me" diatribe is helpful. Later, it reinforces the self-perpetuating grieving behavior so that his need to not improve is stronger than his need to improve, due to the "goodies" received for remaining injured.

Arguing. Making statements like, "Now, don't talk like that! What would … [important person] say if they heard you talking like that?" in response to "I wish I would have died!" simply deny the loss and the magnitude of it. Your survivor can be driven further into depression and suicidal ideation if he is not allowed to express his despair at his losses. He may think, "They don't understand.", "I can't talk to anyone.", and "I feel so alone!"

What to Do

Remind him to get active. Exercise has been proven to relieve stress.

> Honesty is stronger medicine than sympathy, which may console but often conceals.
> — Gretel Ehrlich

Offer understanding. Acknowledge the loss and the struggle to deal with it. Listen with your heart. Say something like, "You have sustained a serious injury and I know how hard it is for you. It would certainly be a lot easier just to quit, and I give you a lot of credit for … instead of…, and I know that you will continue to do your best to…"

Provide perspective. Remind him that these feelings won't last forever, rather than arguing as in the "What not to do" example. Reframe what DJ told me: "Soon you'll find that a part of each day won't be so awful. Then, a bigger part…" See *Brain Injury Rewiring for Survivors.*

Offer verbal support. Because survivors often become more externally driven after the injury, due to diminished self-trust, a vote of confidence by a significant person is powerful. Listening to motivational audio or video tapes may be helpful.

> Sandwich every bit of criticism between two layers of praise.
> — Mary Kay Ash

Personal experience. My father, a former coach, encouraged me with "Do one more than you think you can, Honey" whenever we did something. This was effective for at least two reasons: it placed the responsibility on me to accomplish goals that I set and it demonstrated his confidence in me to do one more — which inspired me to actually do two more!

Offer non-verbal support, such as:

- Hugs and smiles suggest "I'm with you; I care." A touch or squeeze is invaluable.
- Visual reminders, such as cards that express positive messages, can provide a lift. "You're a winner!" and "We're proud of you!" — cards that my folks sent years ago still grace my refrigerator door.
- Silent companionship may sometimes be all that's needed. If someone — anyone! — shows interest and invests time, your survivor feels less hopeless, less lonely, and less depressed.
- Thoughtful use of humor may help some survivors, e.g. funnies, comic/cartoon books, or video/audio tapes.
- Animal-assisted therapy can be especially helpful. Pets not only provide unconditional love, they often sense what to do. Caring for a pet offers diversion and control over something.

Provide opportunities for control and decision-making about certain aspects of his life, such as what and when to eat, or when and if to go somewhere. Ask, "What is the best time for you to do…?" Knowing that he has control over some things in his life leads him to take more responsibility and to feel a sense of mastery in other areas of his life. This kind of power is addicting — in a good way!

Seek community enrichment resources. You and his therapists are not required to provide all the answers. Ask others!

Provide opportunities to deal with anger. Know a variety of anger-defusing activities to have ready for various moods. (See suggestions in the *Brain Injury Rewiring for Survivors*, Emotional Rewiring chapter).

Before an outburst:

- Together, list constructive ways to defuse and redirect his anger.
- Remind him of his list — before he blows up — and then invite him to go with you to safe venting places as you grab soft and safe items.
- Be alert to the warning signs that anger is emerging. He may not be able to feel anger rising or sense other cues in himself before he explodes.
- If you sense an imminent outburst, distract him with an activity or item.

> Expect people to be better than they are; it helps them to become better. But don't be disappointed when they are not; it helps them to keep trying.
> — Merry Browne

When an outburst occurs:

- Engage him in anything physical, creative, or relaxing.
- Comfort him physically.
- Play relaxing music.
- Remove him from the source of stress.
- Ask him what he needs — but note that he may be unable to tell you.

Does he need to vent? Are there safe ways for him to defuse anger?
Yes. When anger is outwardly expressed, it doesn't build internally as quickly or as dramatically. To provide a healthy outlet, invite him to create and destroy things with sand, clay, or another soft medium. Experts find that releases of violence, such as hitting pillows and punching bags, may instead intensify the rage — exactly the opposite effect!

As we can see from this section, grief is a normal process for dealing with loss. It is important for both you and your survivor to go through the process, including dealing appropriately with the anger. Then you can get on with building a new life with what is left.

Substance Use, Abuse, and Treatments

If your survivor used substances before his injury, he's not alone. If you suspect that he's using now, see Treatments later in this chapter.

Use and Abuse

Survivors have been shown to be twice as likely as others in the community — 35% vs. 17% — to have used or abused drugs or alcohol — sometimes both — before their injury (RTC, 2000). And as many as 67% of those in acute rehabilitation had a pre-injury substance use disorder (Corrigan, 2003).

What substances?
Alcohol was preferred by 83% of those injured. More than 50% of survivors had used some marijuana. Beer was the drink of choice for 74% of the imbibers, typical for the population and culture of those most frequently injured — young and male (Corrigan, et al., 1995).

Use patterns post-injury.
Survivors demonstrated troubling patterns:
- Of those who abstained or were light drinkers before injury, 20% began high-volume use after injury.
- Of the pre-injury low-volume users, 36% had increased to medium-volume use at the time of referral. (Kreutzer et al., 1995).
- Regardless of the amount consumed pre-injury, use increased as time after injury increased.
- Medium- or high-volume use was reported by 28% of persons two years or less since injury, compared with 38% in the two- to five-year-after-injury range and 48% of those more than five years after injury (Corrigan, et al., 1995).

Marijuana. The most widespread and frequently used illicit drug in the U.S. — 62 million Americans have tried it at least once — it was used by more than half of the 211 survivors in the Corrigan, et al. (1995) study.

Clinical experience shows that it significantly affects memory and concentration during use and that these effects on memory persist for several days. Connections have been demonstrated between regular use and increased paranoia, as well as being stuck both cognitively and behaviorally. These behaviors naturally cause negative consequences in relationships at school and work and in the family (Corrigan et al., 1995). See *Brain Injury Rewiring for Survivors* Chapter 6 for details of specific effects.

User patterns. Cigarette smokers are five times more likely to smoke marijuana — the link is associative, which means that environmental and social influences can lead to marijuana use. Marijuana is typically combined with other substances, like alcohol and cocaine — combination of substances can lead to the emergency room.

Methamphetamine. This very addictive stimulant drug, commonly known as speed, is ingested by smoking, needle, snorting, or orally. When smoked, it is typically called crystal or ice, which describes the appearance of the clear chunky crystals. When ingested by other methods, the white, odorless, bitter-tasting crystalline powder is easily dissolved in water or alcohol.

Originally used in nasal decongestants and bronchial inhalers, meth increases activity, talkativeness, blood pressure, and heart rate, and decreases appetite. Effects of abuse include irritability, anxiety, confusion, paranoia, aggressiveness, insomnia, tremors, cardiovascular collapse, and death (NIDA, 2007). Be alert to these side effects your survivor could exhibit — meth is becoming the most abused drug in the country. In addition to causing addiction, chronic abuse significantly changes how the brain functions, damaging neuron cell endings and altering the activity of the dopamine system (NIDA, 2006 & 2007).

Cocaine. Most coke users snort this stimulating white powder through the nose; some dissolve it and inject it into a muscle or vein. Smoking crack, a chemically altered form of cocaine, more quickly reaches the brain to produce the most dramatic high — followed by an equally dramatic low.

Reasons to use and abuse. Some researchers suggest that survivors are self-medicating for injury problems. *No kidding! — We survivors feel sad, mad, and/or bad.* Awareness of damage and feeling incompetent are likely reasons many of us go through a stage — long or short — of alcohol and/or drug abuse, either of prescription or street drugs. Your survivor may think, "I'm screwed up anyway, so I may as well totally dilute the pain!"

Physically, he may seek ways to alleviate the constant pain. Emotionally, he's depressed and wants to escape from reality to feel better — even if only for a short time. It's also likely that his grieving has so far been ineffective or non-existent. Mentally, he's aware of few other options or is unable to process what's available. Socially, he probably feels isolated, yet has increased leisure time. Substance abuse provides a more socially acceptable disability than brain injury — and he may lack social expectations for what to do with himself post-injury.

What to do: Whether his injury was use-related or not, inform professionals about any possible substance abuse, so that treatment can be incorporated into his rehabilitation and he can be educated about the negative effects of alcohol and other drugs.

Ask for referrals to alcohol and drug treatment programs, request that he is properly medicated, and watch his behavior for the telltale signs of use. Cognitive-behavioral therapy is especially effective. It identifies and replaces the user's irrational beliefs — "the only time I feel good is when I'm high" — with rational thoughts — "It's hard to learn to be comfortable socially without doing drugs but people do it all the time."

If your survivor was a non-user before his injury, know that he is still at a high risk of developing a substance abuse disorder after his brain injury (RTC, 2000) — and act accordingly!

Treatments

Will he change? — Really? — Good news! If his injury was alcohol-related or he was a heavy alcohol user, he'll be more motivated to change his drinking behavior (Bombardier et. al., 1997). It's not a quick fix, however — he probably didn't start drinking just before his injury and he may need to go through several stages before he's ready to change. Brain injury combined with substance abuse presents a dual challenge — success is dependent upon the Three C's: counseling, commitment, and compliance (To, 2006).

Interventions help with readiness for treatment. A financial incentive proved highly effective for both attendance and successful completion of a program, as did reducing barriers to attendance (Corrigan & Bogner, 2007). While counselors usually tailor treatment to an individual's "stage of change" (Corrigan and Lamb-Hart, 2004), the choice of program is vital — survivors require a different approach and program.

Timing of treatment. Just as survivors who engage in rehabilitation immediately after injury have better outcomes than those who seek intervention later, so do those who begin substance abuse treatment sooner post-injury. Clients who entered treatment during the first three months post-injury were more likely to have maintained abstinence and be engaged either in employment or in productive activity than those who sought treatment later (Corrigan et al., 1995).

Biochemical connection. As vital as your survivor's motivation is, equally important to treatment success are his inherited neurochemical and neurobiological systems. This is because alcohol and drugs' addictive properties are produced by their action on his brain's reward system (Koob, 2006). Low serotonin levels create a brain dysfunction that can lead to alcohol abuse (Lovinger, 1999). If medication raises his serotonin levels, this part of the problem is solved and you can work on the other factors that you can do something about!

Medication treatment. Of the three FDA-approved drug treatments that are currently available, disulfram (Antabuse) causes unpleasant reactions when combined with alcohol, but its use for survivors is discouraged (Corrigan & Lamb-Hart, 2004). Naltrexone (ReVia) blocks the alcohol high, and acamprosate (Campral) reduces craving and relapse drinking by resetting the neurochemical system (To, 2006).

Exciting news! The anticonvulsant topiramate (Topamax) significantly reduces alcohol consumption and improves physical health and quality of life. In a clinical trial of 370 adults, topiramate effectively treated alcohol dependence by reducing the compulsion to drink and improving physical and psychosocial well-being (Johnson et al., 2008). Ask your doctor if it's right for your survivor.

Community-based programs. Of survivors who worked with a team of professionals that provided a systematic approach, 75% were abstinent or had reduced use at one year and 60% were competitively employed or engaged in productive activities (Corrigan et al., 1996).

A team approach is most successful for those who need help to both stop using and start working. Survivors who had already achieved reduction of use or abstinence and were competitively employed were able to maintain both without the team approach (Corrigan et al., 1996).

Treatment results from studies of survivors in substance abuse programs (Corrigan et al., 1995 and 1996) illustrate these factors:

- Positive behavior changes occur: either reduced use or abstinence and increases in productive work or training activity.
- Monitoring (monthly, then quarterly) improves compliance.
- Those who are involved in either productive activity or employment (volunteer or paid) are motivated to both abstain and maintain or to reduce use of drugs or alcohol.

Common to all of these factors is people power — human contact. "Probably the best way to prevent substance abuse following head injury is to ensure meaningful relationships and activities to maximize quality of life...If there are no voids, there will usually be no attempts to fill them with chemicals" (Falconer, 1997).

What you can do. Inform any provider about possible emotional, behavioral, and cognitive problems. Become familiar with the way self-help groups operate and accompany your survivor to the first few meetings to share the experience with him. Be aware that forcing a self-help program on someone who isn't ready is counterproductive.

Consequences without treatment

The costs of not treating those with substance abuse problems are far greater than the costs to treat — for society as well as for survivors and their families.

Income/job loss. Of the 211 survivors in one study, nearly 70% were either not working or in school at the time of referral. This figure reflects a 60% decrease from pre-injury to post-injury productive roles. Even more alarming, of the survivors who were assessed, 82% were not gainfully employed, 41% reported that their primary income was from a government support program, 13% were receiving disability insurance, and 22% were supported by a family member.

Hospital/jail visits: Some survivors love hospitals and jails! For the 58 who were one year or more post-injury, there were 26 emergency room visits and 32 hospital admissions during the previous 12 months. For the 41 survivors who were more than two years post injury, there were 32 arrests in the previous 24 months — half of this group had been arrested at least once! (Corrigan et al., 1995).

Conclusions

Drinkers will continue to drink and other users will continue to use — despite their protests to the contrary — unless and until they are involved in a treatment program. While treatment alone won't make Boy Scouts out of substance abusers or ensure that they stop using and become productive, it promises them helping hands to pursue training, rehabilitation, and employment.

Emotional Issues

To recover from a damaged brain is complicated! Here are some of the emotional reasons:

Failure.

Your survivor may feel that he is not okay because he is not able to do what he could do pre-injury.

Personal experience. For years immediately after my injury, it seemed that I failed at most things I attempted — whether it was at relationships, sports, or jobs — in other words, at life. I'll never forget the day I awoke thinking, "I wonder what I'll discover that I can't do today." I had to face the awful reality that I was not the way I used to be and that I couldn't do what I wanted to do. Because I am known for my tremendous drive — "your greatest strength and your greatest weakness" — that day was one of the worst days of my entire life.

Control and responsibility.

Survivors often feel that everyone is trying to take control from them — where it belongs — and give it to someone or something else. When we who were formerly self-sufficient are told, "Let me handle this. Give me this responsibility. You don't need to worry about it," we feel angry and powerless. The importance to us is illustrated by the following:

Personal experience. One of the events that led to my first suicide attempt was a meeting in which the doctors and my parents decided what to do with me after discharge. Despite an "A" average in graduate school, a teaching career, and thirty years of life, I was not invited to the meeting. Did I feel irate and unimportant!! Although I was injured, I still had the intellectual capacity to understand, and I certainly needed to participate in my own rehabilitation plan!

Note: discharge meetings are different now. Survivors are routinely included. Resuming control and responsibility is a treatment goal.

Clamor control: the nightmare of noise.

Any unpredictable, sudden, and/or loud noise, disharmony, or crowds may be a source of distress. Even formerly ignored or tolerated sounds, e.g., barking dogs, may cause pain now that his "screen" is destroyed.

Yes, he can plug his ears or run away. But the damage is done. Ear-splitting isn't just a descriptive adjective. It's true — these sounds do split us. Our senses reverberate. But unlike Humpty Dumpty, we can put ourselves back together again — it's just not fast. In the meantime, we may regress into childish behaviors like hiding our faces in a pillow. Or we may sob uncontrollably and blame our loved ones for not protecting us. (See *Brain Injury Rewiring for Survivors* for a description of "the leaf blower incident.") While it's difficult to understand his brain pain, consider that whatever he does is his best attempt to cope. It will get better. What to do? Use SAFER and:

- Help him find ways to cope before he blows his circuits.
- Help him to avoid known sources of distress and/or help him leave these places fast.
- Suggest ways to fight back with sounds of his choosing.
- Continue to seek solutions that work for all of you.

The "S" Words: Swearing.

Frequent swearing is another disturbing injury behavior — especially if your survivor rarely or never swore before the injury. His cursing now is almost an involuntary anger response and is probably due to several factors, both directly and indirectly related to the brain damage:

- Increased impulsivity and lack of inhibition.
- Language choice may be instinctive and vocabulary reduced.
- He has fewer alternative behaviors to rely on and a lower stress tolerance.
- He needs a less complex and stimulating environment.

What to do: Help reduce emotional stressors so he stays peaceful. Make a fun activity out of finding other harsh-sounding words or creating nonsense words. Seek ways to enrich his environment.

SSSSSSStuttering.

Survivors who spoke fluently before their injury may stutter or stammer and experience other language problems evident in both expressive and receptive speech, due to the common processing delay. As with numerous other cognitive problems, emotional stress makes it worse.

How to help: Patiently wait for him to finish his sentences. Removing the stress that provoked the stuttering can usually alleviate it.

Self-mutilation.

This phase may be external and intentional or internal and unintentional (poor eating habits). Depending on the psychic makeup of your survivor and where he is in his climb, it may or may not occur. While understandably confusing to you, self-mutilation is similar to the head banging that kids with autism display — for survivors it is an outward manifestation of an irresistible urge to stop what is going on inside our heads: *"If I hit it hard enough or cut it deeply enough or burn it badly enough, maybe I won't feel the pain and it might even go away..."*

__Personal experience.__ I'd revert back to this stage after another social or vocational disaster, usually a combination of relationship collapse and being fired from my job. A favorite spot on my left arm beckoned to me to cut and burn it. The first time, I drew a Jewish star on *my left forearm with a paring knife — not my right arm, because I'm right-handed and not that stupid — and put out 13 cigarettes in the center for a dramatic red-and-black work of art. I did it at night — when all the "demons" appear!*

The next day I ventured down to the clinic where I saw my psychologist DJ, and presented myself to the resident there. He was so alarmed by my casual approach to a serious injury that he wanted me hospitalized immediately. Fortunately, DJ disagreed and I was spared. In our subsequent discussion a breakthrough occurred.

Importantly, DJ didn't ask me why I did it, because I couldn't tell him. Rather, he asked me to describe the design, which was easy. My artwork represented red and black: red for the constant pain and black for the constant hole of despair. DJ helped me understand that I tried to block out the mental pain with the physical pain. When the bodily pain couldn't overpower the psychic pain, I stopped, exhausted at the attempt; once again defeated and bewildered. Once I could label the colors with feelings and attach some rationalization to the deed, I did not feel sick and could begin to understand the meaning of the event.

In addition to exploring the symbolism, we planned how to avert future cuttings and burnings, including exercise, of course! One of his tactics was that I act as co-therapist, meeting with hospitalized self-mutilators whose arms were totally a mass of scars. I decided I did not want to look that way, so worked harder in my twice-weekly therapy.

I'd like to say that the deed wasn't repeated after I left his care. It was, but only three other times and not nearly as drastically. The relapses only involved a knife — I wasn't smoking by then! — and were always circumvented by a visit to the health club where I could engage in a very strenuous workout that caused good physical pain, not damage.

Suicide

Suicide is one of the most important aspects of emotional issues. Your survivor is at risk, but there are things you can do to significantly reduce the risk. While difficult for you to face, your survivor could still lose his life — this time by his own hand. Recent research supports my belief that most survivors attempt suicide in one way or another, at one time or another, at least once. In fact, after release from acute care, suicidal ideation and attempts are common reactions to injury. Realize that most suicidal people do not want death; they just want the pain to stop. The impulse to end it all, while overpowering, is temporary.

How many?
One facility identified 26% of their outpatient survivors as attempters, with 44% of them making repeat attempts (Simpson & Tate, 2005). Another study classified 1/3 of all their TBI patients at clinical risk to commit suicide (Leon et al., 2001).

Who's at risk?
All survivors, especially females and those between the ages of 21 and 60. Additionally, the risk of dying by suicide for stroke survivors is about double that of all other causes (Teasdale & Engberg, 2001). For males, a history of TBI increased the likelihood of attempting (Oquendo et al., 2004). Survivors who both abused substances and suffered emotional disturbance were 21 times as likely to attempt suicide (Simpson & Tate, 2005).

When?
While the greatest risk is the first five years after stroke (Teasdale & Engberg, 2001), the danger actually lasts a lifetime because multiple factors, rather than one or two alone, lead to a suicide attempt (Rudd et al., 2006).

Risk factors.
The injury — whether stroke or mild or greater TBI — contributes directly to suicidal ideation, attempts, and completions. Most significant is a high degree of negative thinking and hopelessness, along with post-injury emotional/psychiatric disturbance. Pre-injury characteristics of those who attempt include depression, substance abuse, hostility and aggression (Simpson & Tate, 2002 and 2005; CAMH, 2003; Teasdale & Engberg, 2001; Oquendo et al., 2004).

Warning signs.
These include an upsetting event, strong emotional state (e.g., anxiety and/or agitation), reckless/self-destructive actions, withdrawal, dramatic mood changes, deterioration in occupational or social functioning, increased substance abuse, preoccupation — talking, reading or writing about suicide or death, giving things away, visiting/calling people to say goodbye, and organizing or cleaning bedroom "for the last time" (Rudd et al., 2006; Suicide Awareness Voices of Education-SAVE, 2007).

Serotonin link.
Low serotonin level has been found to be an indicator of risk for suicide attempts and completions (Knowlton, 1995; Engstrom et al., 1999; CAMH., 2003). Strikingly, 95% of those who commit suicide are found to be deficient in serotonin in certain brain regions (Knowlton, 1995). These regions are in the prefrontal cortex (Arehart-Treichel, 2003) — an area that is commonly damaged in TBIs!

Reasons for contemplating suicide.
Suicidal ideation and amount of preparation is directly related to the lack of success that survivors feel in their lives.

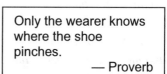

Only the wearer knows where the shoe pinches.
— Proverb

    Depression: "Depression can magnify the rigidity of black or white thinking and can cause people to see all problems as personal, pervasive, and permanent" — the three Ps. (Baser, 1995). They think, "It's all my fault; nothing I do ever works and it's always going to be like this, so I may as well end it all. Everyone will be better off without me and I won't have to deal with this horror show anymore."

    No other options. Due to the brain damage, survivors' problem-solving abilities are reduced. Others are able to confront an obstacle, list options, choose one that makes sense, and act. Survivors lack these skills, especially the "make sense" one. So, unable to seek other workable ways to deal with the pain, the suicide-prone believe there is no other way out.

    Resignation. "Either-or," "black-and-white" thinking leads to the conclusion that the injury was just fate.

Belief in suicide as an "honorable" act. "I no longer bring shame to my family if I'm not here. They have enough trouble without all my problems. I can remove a lot of their misery and make them proud of me at the same time. I can die with honor and bring them peace."

Hopelessness. "All I see is a winding path that goes up a mountain and never comes down. There is no light at the end of the tunnel — just a black hole. Hell, I can't even see around the next bend! It's all up and too high for me to climb now. It's so confusing to never know what I'll be able to do! Some days I can do some things; some days I can do nothing. No one understands this feeling of failure. Others may fail on occasion; I fail frequently. I am not okay and never will be."

Personal experience. I recall some of the events around my first suicide attempt. Interestingly, my shrink at the time gave me the idea when he questioned "whether the accident of a young attractive school teacher was a suicide attempt." — In this case, instead of "Minor Deity," MD stood for "Mighty Dumb!"

About 15 days after the accident I was released from the hospital because they didn't know what to do with me and "there was no reason to keep her."

It is important to note that this was in 1976 — a time when it was assumed there wasn't any damage unless an X-ray showed it. The decision to release me was made despite evidence that I had been unconscious over six hours and exhibited more than a few deficits. To use medical lingo, I presented with receptive and expressive language problems, hemiparesis (one-sided weakness), light-headedness, confusion, visual-perceptual problems, motoric slowing, and internal bleeding from breaking the wooden steering wheel with my chest, bruises from head to knee, and a lot of pain — everywhere.

The act: In keeping with the propriety of the day and my aversion to violence, I made the attempt with various leftover drugs washed down with Chivas Regal. Thanks to all the accumulated medications from attempts to restore my body and mind — from the other accidents, divorce, and loss of my home and school — and the new drugs, there was no problem downing an adequate number to do the deed. In the 1970s, all problems were solved with drugs and more drugs and the theory that "If one drug didn't work, let's change the diagnosis and try another!"

I left the door to my apartment unlocked so my mother, a private person, would be spared the embarrassment of asking the manager to open the door and then finding me dead in the presence of a stranger.

Psychological misinterpretation. *This thoughtful gesture and that I remembered what I drank with the pills were both misunderstood by the drug-pushing shrink I had at the time. Because I left the door open and remembered that I drank Chivas Regal, he decided that I was trying to get attention by my suicide attempt. Hogwash! I tried to kill myself and wanted to go out in style! That someone would care enough to give me such good booze for Christmas made me feel good. That's why I drank that brand — not because I wanted attention.*

Aftermath. *The misinterpretation and subsequent monitoring of all my medications, as well as the search by my parents for any other hidden drugs, served to push me further into despair. I wanted to forget that my brain didn't work, and alcohol — especially combined with other medications or street drugs — was the perfect way to forget. My brain normally forgot a lot, but it didn't forget its incompetence — ever!*

Postscript about suicide "demons." *My suicide "demons" eventually stopped coming. Although they still visited me on occasion for more than 25 years after my injury, they weren't as pernicious and didn't stay as long as in the bad old days.*

Winter, with its early darkness and multiple rainy days in a row that prevented outdoor exercise, brought back the demons. My lack of control over unpredictable emotional storms, combined with the noise from the blustery wind and pounding rain, made me feel especially vulnerable. I dreaded finding the latest leak. But then I'd think, "You could still be stuck in Minnesota — or, God forbid, Texas!" and proceed to clean up the mess.

Typically, it took a combination of inclement weather, the holidays, hitting another wall, and a job or relationship collapse for the demons to return. They seemed to lie in wait for the obstacles to pile up and for me to be worn down!

How did they go away? *I developed more weapons to fight them and stopped hiding them, telling friends when I was in trouble. The key tool* *for demon relief was to use a light box, especially during the winter, when SAD (Seasonal Affective Disorder) is the worst. It now shines brightly during both breakfast and lunch — and I'm much happier all year.*

I also heard voices talking to me: "What will they tell your kids at church — that you quit? — after you told those same kids not to quit when learning to surf? Besides, Marlys told you it would take her 10 years to get over it if you killed yourself. Do you want to do that to her? And quitting makes Rewiring *a fraud! What kind of role model would you be, then? People look to you to be tough."*

So I followed my own advice: "Call one of your friends. Go to the ocean, the gym, for a run, or bike ride. Garden. Play happy music. Read the Bible. Practice yoga. You could even go shopping or clean!"

To protect myself and prepare for them, I also used a strategy to set myself up for success: be on "demon alert" during critical times of illness and inclement weather. The only problem with this plan to be a recluse was that I'm a very social person and people make me feel valuable and happy. But, with demons lurking, I wasn't fun anyway, so I exercised — hard — alone first or went to the ocean. Then I linked with my friends!

Although I needed to be on "demon alert" for over two decades when they haunted me, the tough-love self-talk and the accompanying action worked. I'm now 30-plus years post-injury, planning my triathlon season and vacations, feeling good and generally happy.

What helps?
Experts suggest the following:
- Strong family, friends, faith, and community connections.
- Ongoing medical and mental health relationships.
- Restricted access to lethal means of suicide (guns, knives).
- Easy access to a variety of medical resources and support.

Note: Participants in a cognitive therapy group reported significantly less hopelessness — one of the most prominent risk factors for suicide — and were 50% less likely to reattempt suicide than those in a group with only tracking and referral services (Brown et al., 2005).

What you can do. In addition to following the above suggestions, pay attention to the risk factors and warning signs mentioned earlier. If your survivor is not in immediate danger, acknowledge that the pain is legitimate, that suicidal feelings are temporary, and offer to work together to get help.

If you see warning signs, ask questions about his plan and call someone on your medical team for help. If the crisis is acute, call 911, a suicide or crisis hot line, or take your survivor to a medical facility. **Do not** leave him alone, minimize problems, judge him, or try to shame him to change his mind

Family Rewiring

It's the typical grief scene: First, shock, then denial, followed by worry and confusion — often all of these intermingled.

> Love, love, love!
> — Patricia P. Marshall

"Oh no! My poor..." Then, "Who is this person?" "This is not my son/daughter/husband/wife. This is not my father/mother/brother/sister." "Will he/she be all right?" "What can I do?" "What's going to happen?"

Family dynamics and family challenges.
Because more contacts occur in the family than anywhere else, loved ones also suffer from the survivor's brain injury. That the family members are the true victims of brain injury is a concept shared by many — including experts. And while each individual member may feel the loss in a different way, the family as a system is changed and challenged by the injury. What are the wounds?

Because of your survivor's differences, harmonious relationships are tested. Nothing is the same and never will be again. Previous roles and expectations are no longer valid. Pre-injury abilities may or may not be exhibited again. Your survivor may not even be aware of the differences. Problems emerge.

Family therapy.
"Why did the doctors suggest psychotherapy for the family? We're not injured or crazy — he's the one who needs a shrink! Besides, he's getting

better. Thanks anyway, but we don't need help to adjust. We've been through bad times before. We'll be fine, thank you. Our family can take care of itself."

Maybe — maybe not. You may not know that cognitive and social skills improve more slowly than physical ones — and that this leads to major communication problems.

As with other group conflicts, better outcomes result when members seek solutions together. Research has shown that survivors do best when their families are involved in team treatment, supporting and accepting the survivor and his team, and are realistic about his deficits and outcome.

What happens in therapy?

During meetings with a trained counselor, family members can safely express emotions that they may be unaware of or embarrassed to show. They also learn how to accept and support the survivor, discuss necessary role changes within the family system, and explore possible treatment options. This is a time to problem-solve and agree on solutions as a family.

Why not apply our reliable SAFER method to rewiring the family? You can develop a plan that considers everyone's needs, where the needs of the family as a functional unit are placed above the needs of any member — injured or not — while incorporating the "new" member into the family's old system. Family members can return later to analyze what isn't working, reformulate possible solutions, and agree to try again.

Summary

I hope that the "Emotional Rewiring" for both you and your survivor will flow easier now. Be sure to talk with his medical team because less, more, or different medications or other treatments can alleviate some of the problems he —

> Grief can't be worked out if people don't talk about the person who has died.
> — William Pinsof

and you — experience. If you continue to seek solutions, so will he! Believe that your survivor can rewire successfully — with your help.

Points to remember:
- Understand that trauma reactions are like grief responses.
- Know that his behavior — not him — is at fault.
- Do not accept undesirable behavior.
- Know that rebuilding self-esteem at this stage of life is similar to developing it in his first few years of life.

> Honesty is stronger medicine than sympathy, which may console but often conceals.
> — Gretel Ehrlich

- Seek the help of a mental health professional when your survivor demonstrates depression or aggressive or suicidal behavior.
- Express condolence with a touch, a hug, or just silent companionship — there may be little need for words.
- Consider healing rituals and creating your own memorial rite.
- Allow yourselves to grieve, too.
- Be alert for substance abuse and seek treatment if suspected.
- Help him find ways to cope before he blows his circuits.
- Help him avoid known sources of distress and/or help him exit these places fast.
- Suggest ways to fight back against overstimulation with sounds of his choosing.
- Be alert for self-mutilation and suicidal ideation/intent and seek treatment promptly.
- Remind him to get active. Exercise is proven to relieve stress.
- Offer understanding and listen with your heart.
- Provide perspective and companionship.
- Offer verbal and non-verbal support like hugs and visual reminders.
- Provide opportunities for control and decision-making.
- Seek community enrichment resources.
- Provide opportunities to deal with his anger.
- Your family also suffers, so strongly consider family therapy.

7

Body-Mind Rewiring: Healing with Conventional Medicine

Any path is only a path, and there is no affront,
to oneself or to others, in dropping it if that is
what your heart tells you.

— Carlos Castaneda

"Calling all deities... major or minor ...somebody, please answer..." But whom can we trust and where do we find them? Who and what can switch my survivor on?"

Introduction

Rewiring requires a network of healers. To understand and then decide which treatments to try, you need to know what's available, so this chapter describes many options offered by Western medicine. We investigate new methods that provide new hope, like robot-assisted therapy and neuromuscular electrical stimulation. So you can learn how to obtain the care you seek for your survivor, we talk about self-advocacy with health professionals and medical insurance programs. Personal experience insights that may amplify your efforts are placed throughout the chapter. Conventional medical topics include:

- Depression, psychiatric care, and medications.

- Psychological care — traits of helpful and unhelpful therapists.
- Psychological interventions — EMDR and neurofeedback.
- Vision and vestibular therapy.
- Physical therapy — including new methods such as hippotherapy.
- Recreational therapy — including animal-assisted therapy.
- Expressive arts therapies — art, music, drama, dance/movement.
- Therapeutic devices — light boxes, CES, and TENS units.
- Orthotics and foot dysfunction.
- Medical insurance programs — Medicare and Medicaid.
- Self-advocacy with health professionals.

Psychiatric Care and Medications

Survivor's Depression

"I don't need a shrink and drugs. I'll be fine — just leave me alone!"

Does this sound like your survivor? You're far from alone. Depression is one of the biggest hurdles that survivors and their loved ones face.

Recent research shows that anywhere from 27% to 59% of brain injury survivors experience an injury-induced depression (Seel et al., 2003; Underhill et al., 2003; Jorge et al., 2004). Definitions of depression, sample size, time since injury, and/or methods of gathering data account for the wide variance.

Personal experience. From what I've observed in over thirty years, 100% of all survivors become depressed. Whatever the percentage, who wouldn't feel despair if their whole world crashed?

As discussed in Chapter 6, Emotional Rewiring, it's important to differentiate short-lived depression of mood, which may be caused by loss or disappointment, from clinical depression, which is a prolonged disorder that affects the entire system.

Those diagnosed with clinical depression experience five or more symptoms lasting two weeks or more that are not due to any other physical condition, substance, or medication. See *Brain Injury Rewiring for Survivors* Chapter 7 for symptom information.

The Role of Medication in TBI

The questions and answers in this section are taken from Gardner, 1992 & 2007.

What is included in the evaluation and in a treatment plan?
Biological, psychological, and social factors are all considered. For example, post-traumatic seizures, hydrocephalus, and hypothyroidism are potential causes of depression. Side effects of current medications are also reviewed for potential cognitive and behavioral impairment.

In setting up a treatment plan, we look at problems, possible causes, resources, and unknown factors. Concerns are addressed. We explore the potential usefulness of a spectrum of possible remedies — both traditional and non-traditional — and the risks and benefits of any of our choices.

Why do we use medications? How do they work?
The goal of medication is to empower a person — not to be the power.

The appropriate medication can help to eliminate or reduce problematic symptoms, so your survivor can regain control of thoughts, feelings, and behavior — and use his own efforts to proceed with recovery.

Medications help to correct the balance of neurotransmitters responsible for delivery of signals between nerves so the nerves can fire more accurately. Treating the neurological damage — and thus the organic factors that may predominately cause disagreeable symptoms — effectively removes the static from your survivor's wires. When his brain works properly, he is able to use his psychotherapy sessions to investigate environmental stressors and other attitudes, behaviors, traits, and conflicts that also interfere with his sense of well-being and functioning.

Watch for promising research on medications that can protect nerves from damage and regenerate new brain cells!

Personal experience. *I'm happy to report that treating the neurological damage works! A few years ago an MD suggested that I try gabapentin (Neurontin) for what she called "myoclonus" (mini-seizures). Neurontin stopped the brief shaking I sometimes experienced and fixed*

*my irritable brain with no side effects! I increase the dosage with extra
stress or if I feel agitated and/or depressed. What a miracle!*

What are potential problems/misconceptions with medication use?
To focus exclusively on symptoms rather than underlying problems is a
common and seductive pitfall of medication use. This is like treating a
headache with painkillers while overlooking the underlying brain tumor.

Labeling medications unnatural is also incorrect. Some pharmaceuti-
cal preparations are synthetic copies of natural herbs while others use an
herbal base. Another common misconception is to think of medications
from one of two opposing views, seeing them as a magical cure or
decrying their use as a crutch that indicates a character weakness. Any
"cure" results from a person's actions after the drug removes any
obstructions! It is wise to make use of available crutches to facilitate
repair.

Nor is the role of medication to mask problems and allow your
survivor to passively sit back and let the pills do the work. The biggest
factor in recovery is not medication, but motivation.

How can we avoid medication problems?
- Recognize that some medications, like antidepressants, usually take
  days to weeks to begin to work, and the maximum effect may not be
  felt for more than a month after initiation of a therapeutic dose.
- Consult with your physician if the ratio of benefits to side effects is
  unacceptable. Discuss other treatment options such as changing the
  dose and/or the medication or adding others.
- To prevent over-reliance on medication, you and your survivor need
  to view this intervention as only part of the total treatment program.
  Numerous other therapies require his active participation if he is to
  recover lost skills and learn new ways of adapting.

What are the usual dosage requirements?
To determine dosage standards, manufacturers look at three factors: after
ingestion how much of the drug is absorbed into the bloodstream from
the intestine, how fast is it metabolized (broken down) by the liver, and
how quickly is the drug eliminated from the body through the kidneys or

bile. These factors vary with a person's size, body composition, age, gender, and functioning level of the organs, so an individual dosage level needs to be set. Additionally, because the brain is so dynamic, both psychiatric and physiological changes need to be monitored and dosages adjusted accordingly. Even slight differences in body fluid level and retention affect the blood level of any medication.

Recent research about medications.

Depressed survivors who expect to feel better after taking a placebo (sugar pill) can prime their brains into actually feeling better! Beginning to change the brain pathways with a placebo provides a head start for the anti-depressants that follow and can aid physicians in determining the correct medication.

Regular use of ibuprofen (Advil, etc.) after brain injury worsened cognitive abilities. Researchers found that brain-injured rats whose food contained ibuprofen (proportional to doses taken by humans) performed far worse on learning and memory tasks than injured rats given no treatment at all (Centre for Neuro Skills, 2006). This finding is important for survivors who are typically prescribed ibuprofen or other non-steroidal anti-inflammatory drugs (NSAIDS) on a long-term basis.

For survivors who experience seizures, the anti-seizure medication lamotrigine (also useful for treating Bipolar Disorder because it decreases abnormal excitation in the brain) works for those who did not find relief from mood swings while taking lithium and other drugs (Clinical Drug Invest., 1998; Medline Plus, 2005).

Loved Ones' Depression: What to Do?

Experiencing a degree of depression following your survivor's brain injury is normal, but you don't need to suffer alone — nor is it advisable to do so. While you probably don't need to hear about research studies to convince you of the value of social connections, it is important that you know that research found that caregivers didn't feel distress if they received adequate social support, regardless of the condition of the survivor or the length of time since the injury (Ergh et al., 2002). So, stay connected with your friends, extended family, and religious/community groups — both for yourself and for him. (See the *Brain Injury Rewiring for Loved Ones* Social chapter for more information).

Psychological Care

Once his neurons are better wired, he can "put two words together" — "Boy! Does he need to talk!" Studies show that psychotherapy produces brain changes. Researchers believe changes result from

> Don't push the river; it flows by itself.
> — DJ

an encouraging environment and other positive factors — a good relationship with a therapist, believing and wanting to get better, and hearing that there is hope for improvement (Brink, 2006). *Maybe optimism can cure!*

In my case, the practitioners who helped the most were not conventional in their approach to medicine. In contrast, those least helpful were inflexibly wedded to their dogma and tradition — even attempting to put me in a box — definitely not a good idea! As we all know well, people with head injuries do not fit into a typical anything.

In the many years of receiving talk therapy after my injury, exactly six therapists were significantly helpful to me. Evenly split between men and women, they included two psychiatrists, three psychologists (PhDs) and one MFCC (Marriage, Family, and Child Counselor) intern. All the others, including all other psychiatrists — *apparently I confounded them!* — ranged from somewhat helpful to very destructive for me.

Traits of the most helpful therapists.
- That I had brain damage was believed, with or without evidence.
- We connected. They liked me and showed me respect.
- If I was in bad shape and needed more time, our sessions were extended or extra meetings were scheduled.
- In emergencies, by following our rules I could call DJ at home or page Christine.
- They promptly responded to emergency contact and any other calls.
- They were all highly intelligent and respected my abilities, too.
- They were honest, confronting, and loving — all at once!

- They trusted me and weren't alarmed by anything I did or said.
- They looked at me and responded rather than just taking notes.
- They used a non-conventional approach with a flexible structure.
- We agreed on treatment methods to use and the desired outcome.
- They wanted to learn about me from significant people in my life.
- I found them through a physical ailment (ulcers), traumatic life event (rape, accidents), or the reliving of an awful event.
- The therapists were all within 10 years of my age.
- They referred me to other people and places, and suggested homework.
- We agreed on methods and desired outcome.
- All relationships were long-term — usually two to five years.

Traits of my least helpful therapists.
- I was a patient with at least one disorder — and it varied.
- They could fix it — "Don't worry your pretty little head. I'll take care of it."
- They tried to make me "middle class and normal" — something I wasn't before the injury!
- Their diagnosis kept changing based on the poor efficacy of the medication.
- Medications — emphasis on the plural — were the answer.
- They were very formal and not able to demonstrate caring.
- I didn't feel respected or liked.
- They were impressed with themselves — they were the experts!
- They didn't really believe me or place any value on what I thought was wrong.
- They were unavailable for crisis contacts — too busy!
- They were unprepared for our sessions — *big black mark!*
- They didn't validate or consult me about my goals.
- They acted as though I was "a case" — *not a person!*
- They were not interested in learning anything about me from anyone important to me.
- They refused to help me educate myself about anything related to treatment, e.g. medication side effects or testing.
- They were short-term and we never really developed a relationship.

Personal experience. Suddenly it was slipping again — my elusive sanity, I mean. This time it was shortly after finances dictated a move thirty miles north of San Diego. Without either an MD or therapist I trusted — and after more bad experiences with both — I "let my fingers do the walking" in the psychologists' section of the local yellow pages. What I found was a name I recognized from the San Diego Brain Injury Press, *Christine Baser, PhD — a local clinician recommended by the San Diego Brain Injury Foundation. Was this divine intervention? We met. I liked her. Then I adored her.*

Neuropsychological Care

Shortly after the injury, your survivor will likely link up with a neuropsychologist. These specially trained psychologists evaluate and treat people with brain behavior disorders and examine how the brain injury impacted your survivor's thinking, emotions, and actions.

The scope of the neuropsychologist's involvement may vary from coma stimulation during early stages of recovery to talk therapy later. To help manage agitation, aggression, impulsivity, and other behaviors that may occur, systematic plans are developed with other team members.

A comprehensive neuropsychological evaluation of your survivor addresses what abilities need rehabilitation, how these thinking deficits may affect daily life, and how to prove that cognitive change occurred.

Using insight gained from clinical experience and results from formal test batteries, a neuropsychologist can help you and your survivor identify your survivor's strengths and intact abilities as well as his weaknesses and the severity of those deficits.

Then — on the more personal side — a neuropsychologist can help you and your survivor to understand these mental changes, set realistic expectations for independence and daily functioning, and make short- and long-range plans.

Mindful of injury-caused deficits, a neuropsychologist can work with your survivor to examine how his internal and external environments affect his thinking, feeling, and acting — and how he can obtain and maintain balance. Together, they can explore strategies or adaptations for solutions to specific problems — such as sleep disturbance or poor time management — and to complex problems — such as depression, memory loss, fears, anxieties, and social skill deficits. For example, for noise sensitivity your survivor and his therapist may explore strategies to cope with noisy situations: total or partial avoidance, decreasing or blocking exposure with earplugs or headphones, and/or training to reduce sensitivity to noise.

Broad issues — such as identity, adjustment, family life, and social/ community/vocational re-entry strategies — are also addressed with survivors who develop long-term relationships with psychotherapists.

Those trained in cognitive therapy use special methods to help survivors to reframe, redefine, and revise unhealthy thoughts and beliefs that trigger stress and harmful behavior (Baser, 1998).

Personal experience. Several key links in my rewiring team — including medication management, vestibular treatment, and the use of EMDR (a psychotherapy technique) for relief from noise distress and trauma — were God-sent connections from my beloved Dr. Baser.

Interventions

With the variety of therapeutic options available today, I hope that you and your survivor connect with at least one of these "hot wires."

Eye Movement Desensitization and Reprocessing (EMDR)

EMDR is a non-invasive psychotherapeutic technique that uses a client's rapid eye movements to restore lost balance — permanently and rapidly.

EMDR allows the flow of information processing to continue after a trauma. Processing information requires a balance of excitatory and inhibitory neurons. A trauma produces an over-excitation that disrupts this critical balance and results in overload.

Trauma also stops normal processing and leaves the memory in an anxiety-filled state complete with all the sights, sounds, smells, and feelings of that experience — which may or may not be exaggerated. The clinical term for this is post-traumatic stress disorder (PTSD). Whenever any of the sensory perceptions from the original trauma are present, the painful memory can return. And because a trauma survivor often becomes unusually alert and easily startled, reminders of the event may be everywhere! Life can revolve around reliving the event.

What does EMDR do, how does it do it, and why does it work?
EMDR restores harmony so that the brain waves once again move in synchrony on both sides of the brain. The rhythmic eye movements stimulate the processing system, allowing the memory to remember the event, but disabling and dissipating the associated negative emotions.

Trauma's intensity prohibits normal brain processing and desynchronizes *delta* and *theta* brain waves. Lateral eye movements (saccades) can free the "stuck" effects of trauma, enabling normal neuronal activity to resume so the event can be reintegrated, according to EMDR developer Francine Shapiro, PhD.

EMDR works like dreaming, using the body's natural mechanism of reintegrating and recreating events. Similar or identical to the involuntary rapid eye movement (IREM) that occurs when we dream, these rhythmic eye movements allow the painful memory to be desensitized (Robinson, 1992).

Another theory suggests that a process called "reciprocal inhibition" occurs, in which a relaxation response is paired with a disturbed one, resulting in lessening of the distress (Weil, 1997).

What occurs in an EMDR session?
Under the direction of a trained therapist, a client deliberately retrieves the trauma from memory, complete with the sensory details and thoughts, feelings, and body sensations that accompanied the event. Then the client ranks the intensity of the experience (in terms of anxiety level) on a scale of one to ten. Next, for about 30 seconds, the patient's eyes follow a pen that a therapist rhythmically moves back and forth at a distance of about one foot in front of the patient. Then the client again ranks his level of distress, relates his observations, and refocuses on the event to prepare for the next set of movements.

At the rate of about one cycle per second, a set of 30-50 cycles completes one set. A therapy session may involve only a few or many sets, depending on the discussion in between that is centered on the observations, feelings, and sensations of the client. Relief can be found in one session, and it typically takes ten sessions or less (Robinson, 1992).

If vision is impaired, can EMDR still work? How?

Any kind of rhythmic movements can produce the desired rebalancing. A therapist consults with a client to select the most effective tool (distance from therapist, object, background, etc.) and how to use it. Auditory clicks or physical taps are sometimes used as options to the more typical hand-held pen or finger/hand of the therapist (Bennington, 1997).

What does research say about EMDR?

It works! Recent studies of those who were single-trauma victims demonstrate phenomenal results: after three 90-minute sessions, more than 80% of the study subjects no longer suffered from PTSD — and the cure was permanent! (Bennington, 1997).

Color brain mapping studies of war veterans found that EMDR was seven to nine times more effective than biofeedback and relaxation therapy in reducing symptoms of combat trauma. Want proof? Studies show that trauma halts the synchronized movement of brain waves. And that EMDR treatment frees the brain waves to resume their balanced moves on both sides of the brain (California Psychologist, 1992).

What symptoms will improve? What won't EMDR do?

Trauma survivors of all ages find fast relief from the multiple symptoms of PTSD and other trauma-related conditions, including anxiety, sleep disturbances, flashbacks, intrusive thoughts, concentration difficulties, phobias, relationship problems, and low self-esteem.

EMDR doesn't work like a laser beam to instantly erase bad scars and memories, but it can zero in on the emotional pain caused by the injuries and reduce or eliminate it. EMDR is not a magical cure, but can be used to facilitate the work of trauma relief. Once again, the magic lies in the actions and interactions of the rewiring team — the "reprocessing" — not anyone's magic wands.

Who practices EMDR and whom/where do they treat?

Any mental health practitioner may practice EMDR; official recognition requires the completion of a 35-hour course and supervised practice.

Since EMDR's inception in 1987, 22,000 practitioners now treat people who've suffered physical and/or emotional traumas that range from childhood abuse to sexual assault to natural and man-made disasters.

Accepted by the scientific community after research proved it effective, EMDR-trained teams of therapists treated survivors of such well-known disasters as Hurricane Andrew, the Oklahoma City bombing, Vietnam War, Flight 800 crash-site, and the Los Angeles riots.

Because treatment can trigger intense emotional responses and associations, selection of a trained and empathic therapist is vital. To locate practitioners in your area, contact the EMDR Institute (see resources) or ask one of your rewiring team members.

Personal experience. EMDR worked for me! It's considered to be most effective for survivors of a single trauma — yet my experience verifies that, with the right practitioners, even those of us who've come through multiple traumatic experiences can triumph! I got help from Dr. Christine Baser's colleague Kent Bennington, PhD.

Although trauma resolves faster if treated immediately, when a flashback triggers the experience — as it did for me — the unresolved trauma returns to wreak havoc once again.

Because my auto accident and sexual assault occurred just months apart, seemingly minor events like carpet cleaners mistakenly entering my home, revive the anger, fear, and paranoid behaviors caused by violation that happened 20 years earlier.

Unable to afford a guard dog, I followed the rhythmic pen for a few sessions with Kent as "conductor." He empowered me and restored my usual feelings of imperviousness — and motivated me to place a baseball bat by the door.

Are there other energy techniques like EMDR that seem to work?

One popular method that seems to have effects similar to EMDR is called Emotional Freedom Techniques (EFT). Using this technique the survivor taps with his fingers on locations along acupuncture meridians. The theory is that this releases energy blockages and allows healing energy to flow throughout the body. One advantage of EFT over other energy techniques is that, after learning how to use EFT, your survivor can apply the techniques himself for ongoing issues. There is more information about EFT and how to find a practitioner at www.emofree.com.

Biofeedback

Using lab procedures developed in the 1940s, the Western form of biofeedback enables people to control such supposedly involuntary functions as heart rate, blood pressure, muscle tension, and blood

> Some things have to be believed to be seen.
> — Ralph Hodgson

supply to the skin by using signals from their bodies.

How does biofeedback work?
The biofeedback machine shows changes in muscle activity. Connected by sensors to a device that picks up electrical signals from their muscles, participants see and hear their tension fed back to them from visual and auditory cues displayed on a computer monitor.

Under stress, muscles contract and cause pain. Patients learn to associate sensations in their muscles to levels of tension that are shown in the cues. Slowing down the flashing or beeping signals on the screen requires relaxing tense muscles. With continued training, clients learn to relax muscles at will and thus alter their physiological responses, gradually doing it without the machine.

What conditions of survivors can biofeedback treat?
Anything affected by stress. Importantly for survivors, biofeedback is effective for both tension and migraine headaches, as well as for many other types of chronic pain and for disorders of the digestive and respiratory systems.

Dramatic findings from three states in the US show that some people with spinal cord injuries have regained muscular limb abilities after biofeedback training. Although these results sound miraculous, the reports maintain that the techniques are not new — just a different use.

Neurofeedback

This discussion of neurofeedback is taken from "Neurofeedback as an Alternative Treatment for Head Injury," Dupler, 1998.

What is neurofeedback? How and why does it work?

Neurofeedback is electronic biofeedback — a high tech guidance system for the unconscious mind. It utilizes an electroencephalograph (EEG) machine to continuously measure the quality of neural activity in a specific area of the brain and rewards the client for improvement. Neurofeedback accelerates the rate at which the mind gathers corrective information about itself. When the brain receives reliable information about its shortcomings, it tends to readjust itself to a higher level of functioning rather quickly.

While a computer interprets irregularities in the reading, these findings are presented back to the person in the form of sound, video, or tactile information. Since this feedback information is timed precisely with each error, the mind suddenly has a tangible reference point from which to correct itself.

What disorders and other deficits can neurofeedback help?

Deficits in the EEG rhythms can indicate the presence of such disorders as brain injury, epilepsy, depression, anxiety, and chronic pain. Neurofeedback aids in the proper reorganization of neural pathways and tends to tone and regulate the autonomic nervous system, including the endocrine system. Clients frequently report improvement in secondary symptoms that often occur with brain injury — poor reaction time, inattention, chronic pain, depression, and anxiety. Naturally, this physical and emotional progress further enhances the recovery process.

In addition, neurofeedback has resulted in a 60% to 80% improvement and a significant reduction in medication for those who have used it for Attention Deficit Hyperactive Disorder (ADHD). Similar results were found for those with hypertension (La Fazio, 1997).

How can neurofeedback accelerate recovery from brain injury?
Typically with brain injury, EEG rhythms (brain waves) slow down and diminish in strength at the point of injury, probably due to fewer cells producing neural activity or damaged pathways. Rewarding the production of faster, stronger, and more correct rhythms draws healing attention back to the area. Some lost function may return as the damaged area begins to resonate as it once did. This assists in the reconnection of old neural pathways and accelerates the relearning process.

How successful is it for survivors of TBI? Who improves the most?
In general, neurofeedback will provide some degree of remediation to 80% of TBI survivors. Those who are the most aware and motivated to change will show the greatest improvement. Within the 80% who do show improvement, about one-half will retain the gains made from the initial treatment.

Ultimately, as we all know, recovery from TBI or any brain disorder requires commitment and proactive participation in one's own treatment. This is the beauty of neurofeedback — it is noninvasive and empowers the survivor to take control of the healing process.

How do we select a practitioner? How many treatments are needed?
The practice of neurofeedback requires no special license in most states at this time, so select a practitioner approved by the Biofeedback Certification Institute of America or the Association of Applied Psychophysiology in electroencephalography. Because a biofeedback practitioner may or may not be skilled in neurofeedback, make sure your provider has been trained in EEG neurofeedback and utilizes the latest treatment protocols.

Successful treatment is dependent on a number of variables, but some degree of symptom control is usually found within seven sessions. To attain any permanence, at least forty sessions will be necessary.

Vision Therapy

Not only are eyes the mirror of the soul, they are the primary portal to the world and a barometer of total health. So, considering the many systems affected by brain injury, is it any wonder that the visual information processing system is on the list? Survivors often experience impaired visual perception, which affects their ability to maintain their balance, as well as blurry vision, double vision, and light sensitivity.

Why is a comprehensive visual system evaluation important?

Many motor difficulties naturally result from optic damage. And, because visual pathways also provide from 75-90% of all classroom learning experiences, impaired visual function also affects professionals' assessments of behavioral, psychiatric, and cognitive areas. Survivors may also unknowingly compensate, be unaware a problem exists, not complain, or simply be unable to explain the difficulty (Gianutsos et al., 1988; Valenti, 1998).

What specialists need to be consulted?

Examination for optic nerve damage by an ophthalmologist is warranted because frontal and supraorbital impacts can produce visual difficulties, regardless of the severity of the injury.

Also important in assessment of visual functioning is a thorough optometric evaluation and subsequent treatment. When rehabilitative optometrists worked with cognitive rehab therapists, information flow was greatly improved and treatment compliance was better (Gianutsos et al., 1988).

What assessments and treatments are used for visual disorders?

Different techniques are used, depending on the diagnosis. For example, to identify those who may need special lenses, prisms, or mirrors, an optometric evaluation includes the use of special equipment.

Visual interventions and treatments include patches, injections, and surgery. Obviously, the first choice is the least invasive and most cost-effective modality. Assessment for surgical intervention is recommended no sooner than twelve months after injury to allow for spontaneous healing.

To preserve normal binocular vision, the preferred treatment is to use special lenses rather than an eye patch. Lenses may be rose- or blue-tinted, depending on the needed correction to rebalance the central and peripheral visual systems (Zasler, 1992).

Therapy goals may include returning full visual function, learning compensatory practices (such as how to use special prisms and mirrors), and modifying the environment. For those injured in accidents, therapeutic reliving of the trauma may be included in the behavioral aspects of vision therapy because both physical and emotional traumas affect light perception (Valenti, 1998).

How effective is vision therapy for survivors?

In a study of survivors of severe injuries who were residents of a long-term facility, all who received rehabilitative optometric services benefited and in most cases they participated more in the overall rehab program (Gianutsos et al., 1988). To generalize these findings to other less severely injured survivors seems reasonable and also shows tremendous promise, yes!?

Other balance disorders.

In addition to visual disorders that affect balance, survivors may experience a vestibular (inner ear) disorder. Most survivors of any degree of head trauma experience balance problems. Nearly all moderate injuries and 50-75% of mild injuries cause vestibular dysfunction, which may persist for up to five years. Temporal bone fractures (22% of skull fractures) often result in vestibular nerve lesions. Cranial nerve dysfunction is quite common following brain injuries of any level of severity (Gizzi, 1995).

What are common vestibular disorders?

In addition to reduced balance, the most common vestibular disorder following head trauma is Benign Paroxysmal Positioning Vertigo (BPPV). The primary symptom of BPPV is a spell of violent vertigo that lasts 30 to 90 seconds and is brought on by the typical position of reclining with the head to one side. Many variations of vertigo exist, but those who experience head trauma usually experience vertigo as a false sense of motion, like spinning. Others may feel themselves falling, rising, and rocking.

Does my survivor need to see a specialist?
Yes, because harm may be subtle and symptoms vague, as is common with many residual effects of brain injury. Thus, a cursory exam by a generalist is not likely to detect causal factors for the seemingly minor damage, particularly if your survivor is lying down. Correct detection and diagnosis often requires movement on the part of the injured person.

What kinds of assessments are used for these disorders?
Tests conducted by specialists in auditory disorders such as otolaryngologists include an examination of all systems that contribute to balance and equilibrium maintenance. Thus, visual, auditory, and rotational-movement measurements are taken to detect whether the dysfunction is unilateral, bilateral, or central. Lengthy questionnaires focus on specific symptoms (headaches, dizziness, falling tendencies, clumsiness, speech and hearing difficulties, numbness, etc.).

To evaluate vestibular function, tests may include electronystagmography (ENG) in which an electrical device measures voluntary and involuntary eyeball movements. Another delightful measurement is called a dynamic petrography, in which the patient is rotated after water of various temperatures is syringed into both ear canals to observe fluctuations in the person's center of gravity. Different trials measure fluctuations with eyes opened and eyes closed.

Personal experience. Warning! I could also label this section "How fast can you get sick? Is it cold water or warm water in the ear canal that results in quicker regurgitation?"

What is the principle of vestibular rehabilitation?
Vestibular rehabilitation is an exercise-based approach designed to promote brain compensation for deficits of the inner ear. To remediate disequilibrium and dizziness, therapists direct patients through specific exercises designed to decrease dizziness, increase balance function, and increase general activity levels so that survivors can maintain their center of gravity, regardless of the source of the problem (Shumway-Cook, 2003).

What kinds of therapy are used for vestibular disorders?
Therapeutic approaches are specific to the disorder, although balance training aims to help you survivor maintain his center of gravity, regardless of the source of the problem.

For survivors with the previously mentioned disorder known as BPPV, several positioning techniques known as liberatory movements are used. Balance retraining is a common approach for those with bilateral peripheral disorder and is also helpful to improve stability for people with other balance disorders. Gait retraining is also used. Medications, such as vestibular suppressant medication, were not helpful except to suppress vomiting during the liberatory maneuvers! (Gianutos et al., 1988; Gizzi, 1995; Shumway-Cook, 2003).

Who benefits from vestibular and vision training?
Anyone who experiences difficulties with balance may benefit from professional intervention in both areas. Many problems with balance, coordination, attention, concentration, reading, and other cognitive and functional areas frequently experienced by survivors can often be attributed to eye movement disorders that result from nerve damage to either cranial or optic nerves or both.

How effective is vestibular therapy? Where is help available?
It works! Those with clearly defined peripheral vestibular disorders especially benefit, such as survivors with BPPV who showed a 64% to 100% cure rate! Everyone exhibiting symptoms of dizziness and disequilibrium reported significant improvement (Gizzi, 1995; Shumway-Cook, 2003).

Altering sensory input and other kinds of vestibular stimulation (e.g., body rotation) also improved both the attention span and motor speech performances of survivors with dysarthria and behavior problems (Engberg, 1989).

Additionally, perceptual training improves driving performance. A small group of survivors of brain injury trained with simple paper-and-pencil exercises for 8-10 hours demonstrated increased perceptual skills that also transferred to driving performance (Sivak 1984).

Physical Therapy

Physical therapists play a vital role in rewiring, using various modalities including their hands, ice, and heat to help your survivor learn how to use his changed body. They design programs that use various kinds of equipment, water, and animals to help him improve his ability to function. If he demonstrates paralysis of one or both sides, visual impairment, poor balance, inability or difficulty walking, or general deficits in functional independence, physical therapists can help!

If your survivor works hard, he can increase his physical strength, flexibility, balance, movement, and cardiovascular endurance. And, with those gains, his ability to function improves. That means feeling better and having greater confidence and more independence.

What kinds of goals can we set?

In addition to the areas listed above, goals can include learning how to adapt his environment (wherever it may be), as well as learning how to use adaptive devices. You and other family members can also receive training to work with your survivor to best achieve his goals.

Even if paralyzed, your survivor can become more independent, feel better, and be more in control when he strengthens what remains and learns how to compensate for what is lost. With effort and perseverance your survivor can achieve his goals, set new ones, and keep progressing — I promise!

How does he improve his balance and movement?

Your survivor needs to feel what balance is before he can improve it. Because motion requires spatial awareness and balance, any perceptual and vestibular disorders need to be addressed.

To restore his communication system requires reestablishing the correct muscle firing sequences, which may require mechanical stimulation. Physical therapists may use special stretching methods to rewire the circuits needed for movement. One technique that practices timing the movements of our balance sensors is called proprioceptive neuromuscular facilitation (PNF). Electrical stimulation and biofeedback are also used to restore the timing and sequencing between signals. The practice of cross-body techniques (such as cross-crawling and sliding) to reeducate limb coordination is common. Gross motor games (such as catching a large ball, throwing beanbags, maneuvering an obstacle course, Velcro catch or darts and ring toss) are also helpful. Encourage him to try everything — no matter how silly it seems. With assistance and practice, he can rewire his system.

Recent studies of three new ways to regain use of a damaged limb.
Great news! Limbs damaged by brain injuries can function again using new robotic devices, a muscle-stimulating device, and/or a special intensive therapy method. Again, what we're seeing are "plastic" changes in the brain — new connections form between neurons or existing connections are strengthened — allowing movement to occur!

Increased use of his limbs leads to improvements that are obvious and encouraging for everyone. Strengthening your survivor's affected limbs and improving his motor function leads to greater self-confidence and independence — and happiness!

Robotics to the rescue! New hope for all survivors! One device, worn as an arm brace, works by sensing weak electrical activity in survivors' muscles and providing just enough assistance for them to complete simple exercises (like lifting boxes or flipping light switches). Other devices that can be strapped onto a wrist, hand, or ankle do not take cues from electrical muscle activity but depend instead on the observed motion (or lack of motion) of a survivor's limbs, which means that they can be used by those with no electrical activity in a paralyzed limb.

Survivors who exercised with the arm brace for 18 hours over about six weeks experienced a 23% improvement in upper extremity function (Stein et al., 2007). After gaining FDA approval, the device will be available soon, likely by the time *Brain Injury Rewiring* is published. Even if these robotic devices don't permanently restore lost function, they can be useful as a "power assist" to wear daily (Schaffer, 2007).

How about a hot-wire act to rewire an affected limb? Research found that electrically stimulating an injured arm helps it to move. Called neuromuscular electrical stimulation (NMES), this self-administered therapy uses a device attached to the affected arm to both measure brain impulses and send additional stimulation to aid movement. Survivors watch a visual display to see brain activity related to the muscle and note the threshold line needed to activate the electrical stimulation, receiving both visual and sensory feedback vital to relearning the movement.

Study participants improved strength, flexibility, range of motion, and general motor function, while spasticity and tone were reduced after using the NMES device. Stroke survivors (ages 30-78) used FDA-approved units attached to the arm with electrodes for 20-minute daily intervals totaling about 60 hours over three weeks in home programs. In addition to functional improvements, this study's findings are significant for several other reasons: time since stroke did not impact effectiveness; results were independent of age, side, and nature of stroke; and improvements were maintained long-term. This research was based on a model approved for use in 1997; an upgraded unit is now available (Kimberly et al., 2004; Medline Plus, 2004). See Resources.

How about constraint-induced (CI) movement therapy?

This approach to movement rehabilitation restrains the "good" limb in order to strengthen the affected one. The stronger arm is held in a sling or mitt for 90% of the waking hours over a period of two to three weeks, while intensively training the weaker arm. Intensive daily therapy sessions of six to eight hours are augmented by home practice. Naturally, those who work the hardest show the greatest improvement (Taub et al., 2001; Shephard, 2000; UAB Health System, 2003).

CI creates "rewiring" in the brain because a larger part of the brain is involved in producing movement of the weaker arm after treatment than before. The key is repetition, called "mass practice," that provides stimulation to the previously unused area of the brain, forcing it to reorganize, as it once again receives signals from the affected arm. This triggers new connections (Shephard, 2000; UAB Health System, 2003).

"What? My survivor is supposed to gain movement by restricting it?" Right! While "holding back" part of the body after injury seems counterintuitive, restraining a stronger component requires the weak part to work harder to catch up because it can't borrow strength from the stronger part (Shaw et al., 2003).

When people are first injured, there is a strong tendency to not use the impaired limb. CI therapy overrides this "learned non-use" because concentrated therapy spurs the brain to reorganize and allow an injured limb to regain the ability to function. It's our same use-it-or-lose-it paradigm! (Shephard, 2000; UAB Health System, 2003).

What are the results? Stroke survivors averaging 4.5 years post-injury showed large to very large improvements in the functional use of their affected arm in their daily lives after CI therapy! Significantly, these changes persisted over the two years of testing (Taub et al., 2006). Researchers found that this technique — and its results — also apply to survivors of TBI! (Shaw et al., 2003).

How can my survivor obtain physical therapy (PT) services?
Your physician will write a prescription and refer him. An individualized PT program will focus on the goals determined by your referring doctor, so be prepared to ask for a prescription that covers a broad area! Periodically, your survivor will undergo PT reevaluation. If he demonstrates progress, treatment normally continues, providing your insurance covers it. Note that a written prescription from your survivor's physician is required for all PT services.

Aquatic Therapy

With the guiding hand of a physical therapist in a warm-water pool, your survivor performs various bodily movements, like walking. The water's buoyancy helps to support your survivor's weight, which makes it easier to exercise — and more fun!

In addition, with the resistance from water, he can strengthen muscle groups in ways not available on land. Exercising in warm water also relaxes and massages his muscles, increasing blood flow to injured areas. And, when others are working on their programs, the experience feels more like fun and less like work!

Hippotherapy (Therapeutic Horseback Riding)

This was first used in Europe following two epidemics of polio after World War II. With the similarity of gaits, it's natural to use a horse to treat people with movement disorders.

What kinds of disorders are treated and what are typical goals?

Hippotherapy is recognized as a very successful treatment for such neurological and neuromuscular conditions as traumatic brain injury, cerebral palsy (CP), and multiple sclerosis (MS).

For those with CP, typical goals are to normalize muscle tone and strengthen postural muscles, which increase the ability to perform functional activities of daily living. In addition to improving strength, balance, and coordination, participants gain increased confidence, self-esteem, improved communication skills, and — my favorite — motivation.

What typically occurs in a therapy session?

To optimize the benefits from the horse's movement, a rider is placed in different positions on the horse during a thirty-minute therapy session. Then, while on horseback, the rider performs therapeutic exercises and plays games, based on needs and goals. Each session is directed by a licensed therapist who, in turn, is assisted by an experienced horse handler and volunteer "side walker" (NCEFT, 1997).

Where are rehabilitative horseback riding programs located?

One nationally recognized program, Hope Therapy, is the cornerstone of Moody Gardens on Galveston Island. Formed by a survivor and a son of a foundation trustee after they discovered the healing powers of animal-assisted therapy, Hope Therapy offers hippotherapy to disabled or injured clients ages 14 months to 96 years.

Recreational Therapy

Animal-Assisted Therapy

Animals make therapy fun! Besides providing enjoyment and motivation, they also play an integral role in helping to improve survivors' skills. For example, someone who needs to work on balance and memory may direct his accompanying helper dog in a series of steps and turns. To work on speech improvement, dogs can be trained to respond only to a clearly spoken and correct command. While

> He/she lowers blood pressure, reduces stress levels, decreases depression, increases physical ability, builds self-esteem, and plays one mean game of fetch.
> — Chenny Troupe

commands require clear speech and proper sequencing, negative feedback is limited to a lack of response by the animal — which is easier on the psyche than correction by a human! Rewarding correct performance of a desired task by a dog enhances cognitive skills because attention is required. And manual dexterity improves with other care and feeding chores, like buckling a collar (McLaughlin, 1996).

Although they most commonly provide psychotherapy and physical rehabilitation, occupational therapists (OTRs) also incorporate certified volunteer handlers and animals into their work, adding variety and fun to the often-tedious teaching and learning of necessary self-care tasks.

What are the advantages of using animals?

Besides their role in therapy settings, animals can also help after therapy is completed. Happier and more independent lives for survivors are possible when an animal acts as an incentive to more fully engage in activities. Strangers who would not even think of approaching someone with a disability will pet a dog or pig or stroke a cat or rabbit accompanying a person with a disability — regardless of what the person looks like — since the focus moves from the person to the animal.

What are the benefits of animal-human interactions?
Beyond the physical, social, and emotional benefits that animals provide, they facilitate breakthroughs with certain patients who are unresponsive in other areas of rehabilitation (Voelker, 1995).

And — a medical rarity! — only good side effects result! For example, social therapy dog visits led to significant emotional, physical, and/or social skills progress in over 55% of severely disabled students in special education classrooms in one recent study (McLaughlin, 1996).

Pioneered in 1969 by Boris Levinson, Pet-Assisted Therapy is believed to work because of the "three Cs" — contact, care, and communication between animals and willing humans. And, what can match animals' spontaneous expression of unconditional love?!

Animal-Assisted Activities

While visits by animals to people in hospitals, convalescent homes, homeless shelters, and other institutions are not officially considered therapeutic, their socialization value definitely is! The Animal-Assisted Activities (AAA) program is designed to provide opportunities for human-animal interaction, providing educational and motivational benefits while reinforcing a valuable bond at the same time. Programs include:

Pet partners: Humans and their domesticated animals who are trained to visit people in various settings. Your survivor may be interested in working in this program.

Pets-At-Home: Dogs are most often used, both because of peoples' familiarity with them and because of their abilities.

Assistance dogs include service dogs, hearing dogs, or social dogs. Service dogs can push elevator buttons, turn lights on and off, retrieve items, push wheelchairs, and open doors as they help their owners perform the activities of daily living (ADLs) required to live independently. Dogs can be trained to help pull people out of bed and chairs and help balance them to walk (Wilson, 1993). Hearing dogs alert people with hearing impairments to crucial sounds such as telephone, alarm clock, smoke alarm, baby's cry, traffic, and streetlights.

How does my survivor obtain an assistance dog? What is the cost?
Because of the rigorous screening and training process, patience is required — it could take up to two years to obtain a canine companion. Another option is to train the dog yourself as some people do — a woman with MS trained her dog to load the clothes dryer and fetch things like cash from the ATM machine! (Skenazy, 1993). For those with disabilities, there's no charge! Even though trained canine companions cost more than $10,000 to breed, train, and place, only application and registration fees are required (McLaughlin, 1996).

Animals in Dental Care

Animals also assist dentists. Fish tanks offer a physically relaxing and aesthetically pleasing distraction for anxious dental patients. A savvy dentist and personal attention to mouth care is also an essential part of the entire treatment plan, as the following story illustrates.

> *Personal experience. Watch your survivor's spit production! Without saliva, bacteria thrive. My pre-injury, nearly cavity-free mouth now sets off metal detectors in airports! Why? Four root canals, numerous crowns, and an implant make my mouth more valuable than my auto. It is likely that most of the dental problems were caused by the mouth-drying effect of all the antidepressants I'd taken — without compensatory fluid replacement. So, to prevent this, talk to your health care professionals, take your survivor to visit his dentist, and be sure he can spit!*

Speech-Language Therapy

As key members of the rehab team, these professionals conduct individual and group therapy sessions that forge new cognitive connections and also augment social skills. (See *Brain Injury Rewiring for Survivors* for a personal story.)

> Meet the disease at its first stage.
> — Persius

Occupational Therapy

Working primarily with upper-body deficits, Occupational Therapists (OTs or OTRs) construct braces, splints, and whatever may be needed to enable your survivor to function better in his daily life. They can even visit your home to recommend adaptations to your surroundings. Often, adding adaptive equipment (such as bathroom and hall railings, shower seats, and different light switches, handles, knobs, etc.) makes the difference between your survivor living at home or in an institution. They can also recommend electronic gadgets to keep you all wired!

Expressive Arts

In Spiritual Rewiring, you and your survivor learned how to heal yourselves through music and the arts. Physiologically and emotionally, the expressive arts cause our autonomic nervous systems to produce brain wave patterns that enhance learning, creativity, and dreaming. This inner world of imagery, emotions, visions, and feelings frees your survivor's own inner resources and allows his immune system to operate optimally — to heal him. This section explores how specialists employ the arts in psychotherapy to access your survivor's emotions, empower his inner growth, and help him heal.

Who benefits from expressive arts therapy?

Whether your survivor's choice is music, drama, or a visual or physical art form, expressive therapies offer options for everyone, young or old, large or small — irrespective of disability.

> When words fail, music speaks.
> — Hans Christian Andersen

While helpful for anyone, creative arts therapies are especially beneficial for those who are non-verbal or who do not understand talk-therapy for a variety of reasons — as well as for people who are highly intellectualized or do not speak English at all. Whether your survivor communicates with difficulty or isn't particularly talkative, physical expression provides many benefits that may be unreachable through other methods.

Images are often easier to talk about than vague feelings. And creation of a tangible product — with or without emotional disclosure — is a satisfying experience. Music and art act as vehicles to break through emotional barriers and allow access to painful feelings that your survivor can work through in a therapeutic environment.

Art Therapy

As a non-verbal psychotherapy, art therapy is both diagnostic and healing. Your survivor's creations may symbolize his inner world, ease verbal communication, or merely serve as an outlet for feelings. The art he produces can also serve as a visible representation of physical and emotional growth and healing.

Music Therapy

As a natural healer, music is unmatched. But its magic as a healing tool wasn't "official" until the post-World War I and II eras, when community musicians were hired by hospitals to play for recovering veterans. Their positive response led to the development of the first music therapy program at Michigan State University in 1944.

> I regard music therapy as a tool of great power in many neurological disorders...because of its unique capacity to organize cerebral function when it has been damaged.
> — Oliver Sachs

Music therapy uses music to address the physical, emotional, cognitive, and social skills of people of all ages. In a group setting, participants may play instruments, sing, or just move to music to improve skills and regain their health. Those who can't ordinarily talk or move are often able to sing, and sometimes even dance, to music.

Music therapists also design musical experiences to move participants to deeper states of consciousness. Special vibrations of music and sounds direct their inner journeys, facilitate movement, and enhance physical rehabilitation to meet their therapeutic goals.

Used as a reward in some behavior and biofeedback programs, music's sound and imagery can play an important role in assisting clients to achieve such goals as relaxing a specific muscle group. Music therapists offer both individual and group practice in a wide variety of rehabilitative, educational, and community settings (AMTA, 2007).

Drama Therapy

Acting out feelings may appeal to those survivors who find it difficult to talk or create art. Also termed "psychodrama," therapeutic theater offers a fresh and sometimes funny view of potentially painful thoughts, feelings, and past events under the watchful eye and direction of a skilled drama therapist.

Movement/Dance Therapy

Your survivor will love moving to music or mimicking animals in this therapy! Whether structured or free, physical expression challenges his mind and body to explore feelings kinesthetically and differently than is possible with the other creative arts.

Personal Therapeutic Devices

Several devices help with rewiring, including light boxes, cranial electrical stimulation, and nerve stimulation units.

Light Box

Treat depression, balance brain waves, and reduce pain electronically — without drugs or surgery — thanks to advances in today's technology! Light boxes are one of the best-documented modalities for successful non-invasive treatment of depression. To treat depression with a light box may seem far-fetched, but not if we consider that inadequate exposure to light may cause depression.

What is the role of light?

Essential for our physiological and emotional health, light influences critical aspects of brain function and chemistry, such as regulating circadian rhythms. For example, we're drowsy in the evening because darkness permits the production of melatonin. When light reaches the brain through the retina of the eye, melatonin production stops, explaining why the hormone is used to treat jet lag.

What are our daily light needs and who's light deprived?
For our circadian rhythms to remain balanced, our bodies need 30-120 minutes of natural or artificial light (about 2500 lux — lux is a measure of light intensity). Outdoors on a sunny day, light may reach 100,000 lux, while indoor lighting ranges from 100 to 800 lux — considered "biological darkness" by the brain.

Millions of people are light deprived. Whether they suffer from full-fledged seasonal affective disorder (SAD) or a milder version (winter blues), the cause is the reduced amounts of natural light that fall and winter bring. The incidence of SAD, now officially called circadian rhythm desynchronization, rises with the geographic latitude. In addition to residents of northern climates, shift workers, airplane travelers who cross several time zones, and people who overdose on melatonin supplements are also affected (*Health Confidential*, 1996; Tufts, 1994; Harvard, 1995).

What are symptoms of circadian rhythm desynchronization?
Besides depression, inadequate light has been linked to several other health problems: sleep disturbances, gastrointestinal and menstrual problems, continuous fatigue, sadness, anxiety, social withdrawal, difficulty concentrating, and lack of activity and productivity. Light deprivation is also linked to heart disease and may be a factor in other significant disorders, like breast cancer (*Health Confidential*, 1996).

How is SAD diagnosed? What are the treatment solutions?
Connect the onset of depression with at least two episodes of depressed moods in the fall and winter and non-depressed moods in spring and summer. Eliminate other causative factors, like lifestyle or work-related problems (Tufts, 1994). For survivors, it's the brain injury!

For those who feel slight symptoms of the winter blues, increase exposure to natural sunlight (such as 30 minutes per day outside) and work near a window or in a well-lighted room.

The light box works to reduce depression. In addition, if used every day it can lead to stable sleep and appetite, improved productivity, and better overall health. Typically, light boxes are fitted with a set of two or four non-UV "natural spectrum" fluorescent lights that are attached to a metal reflector and protected with a plastic screen in an approximately eight-pound 12"x24" wooden box (*Health Confidential*, 1996; Tufts, 1994; Harvard, 1995). Newer versions offer LED bulbs. Some boxes use a timer for a wake-up device.

What does research say about light boxes?
Studies since 1985 support claims that light boxes work as a treatment for depression. Scientists who investigated dietary habits of a group of Swiss people found that when those who ate more than one portion of a sweet food in the later part of the day found quick relief from their depressions with light therapy, their consumption of sweets also decreased. Why? Scientists speculate that light triggers the release of the same mood-altering substances that sweets do (Tufts, 1994).

What's the suggested light therapy protocol?
- Use the light box every morning for 30 minutes to 2 hours from October to March (or as many months as needed).
- Sit three feet from the light box (this provides 2500 lux).
- Glance at the light at least once every three minutes while eating breakfast, reading, etc.
- Consult your physician and/or light therapy experts about questions.
- Keep records of sleep, mood, and appetite patterns.

Note: Light therapy does not replace psychotherapy or medications — it reduces the need to increase other treatments during low-light months!

Personal experience. To treat SAD symptoms, I've used a light box during low-light days ever since 1990. Despite living in San Diego, I received less than the amount of natural daylight that my body craved. Medical specialists recommended a light box to treat both the depression and the PMS that blessed me. Another benefit of the light box was that I could keep the same low Prozac dosage winter or summer, rather than

needing to double or triple it in the winter. I've since exchanged Prozac
for a Cranial Electrical Stimulation (CES) device, so now electronics,
rather than drugs, keep my brain working.

Cranial Electrical Stimulation

While this may sound like another insult to your survivor's brain, a CES
unit emits only a tiny amount of electricity and delivers a large benefit!

Cranial Electrical Stimulation can effectively relieve depression,
anxiety, insomnia, phobias, addictive disorders, and hypertension — as
well as chronic and dental pain (Klawansky et al., 1995; Kirsch & Smith,
2000).

What is a CES unit? How does it work? Is it safe?

Palm-sized and weighing 5.5 ounces, a standard CES unit delivers about
100 Hz current at a very small wattage (0.00054 Watts). Powered by one
9V battery, the current delivers an electrical stimulation to the brain
through electrodes that are affixed to the skull in several ways.

CES researchers believe that specific electronic frequencies directly
stimulate the brain's limbic system, the hypothalamus, and/or the
reticular activating system. This action is thought stimulate the
manufacture of neurohormones that affect mood, emotions, and cognitive
abilities, inducing an alert yet relaxcd state that psychologists call an
alpha state (Kirsch & Lerner, 1998; Paros & Kirsch, 1996).

With such a low current, CES units are safe with no known contra-
indications. Naturally, talk with your survivor's physician about his other
treatment modalities because other electrical devices such as pacemakers
and medications that are designed to block neurotransmitters would
interfere with the CES. Increased blood flow to the brain may result in a
slight headache that can be alleviated by reducing current output (Paros
& Kirsch, 1996).

What does research say about the efficacy of CES?

Based on an extensive literature review, positive outcomes were reported
in 91% of the 86 pivotal scientific studies of CES and in 85% of the 40
supporting scientific studies (Kirsch, 2002).

Far removed from the use of electric eels two centuries ago to relieve pain, physicians first reported experimenting with applying low intensity electrical stimulation to the brain in 1902, calling it electrosleep because of its ability to induce relaxation.

Building on the work of scientists from the Soviet Union who treated anxiety with CES during the 1950s, a recent review of studies stated that "it is clearly proven to be the most effective and safest method of treatment for anxiety and anxiety-related disorders, as well as highly effective for depression and insomnia" (Paros & Kirsch, 1996).

Increases in cognitive function and psychomotor abilities also occur (Kirsch & Lerner, 1998). Significant gains on all measures of brain function were found in those treated with the CES unit for chemical dependence and cognitive brain dysfunction (Schmitt et al., 1984).

What is the cost of CES units?
Considering that CES replaces medications, the savings are substantial. Most units cost $200-$500 and are available over the counter, although a prescription is required for insurance coverage. Medicare and many insurance companies cover them. They can be rented from manufacturers and some companies also offer pre-owned units.

Personal experience. I have happily used my CES "brain tuner" ever since the fall of 2001. That previous summer I stopped the Prozac regimen that had worked for ten years because I didn't like the side effects of the sleeping aids that were necessary to counteract Prozac's stimulation. I felt increased anxiety, but wanted a different treatment than medication to control my symptoms. I asked Nathan Zasler, MD, for advice because I respected his work with brain-injury survivors. He recommended the Soto Brain Tuner from Dynamind. It works!

Nerve Stimulation Units

Your survivor can safely manage his pain without popping more pills! Interferential and transcutaneous electrical nerve stimulation (TENS) units can reduce his discomfort when and where he chooses.

The units are palm-sized, battery-driven devices that deliver electrical stimulation to four electrodes that are attached to the body at fleshy locations. The sensation created by the unit works to prevent pain signals from reaching the brain. Though pain relief varies, in many cases the stimulation greatly reduces or eliminates the pain sensation.

How are the electrode sites selected?
To determine optimal site placement, a therapist considers accessibility and proximity to pain and nerve sites. Then electricity is channeled to pain-relief sites through electrodes placed above and/or below, across from or on two sides of, specific pain locations. These points are frequently found in the same location as acupuncture, trigger, or motor points. In fact, research studies found that the actual anatomical and clinical correlations between trigger and acupuncture points is very high (Mannheimer, 1980).

The location of sites greatly impacts the success of the units. If relief is not felt, finger pressure can also locate optimal (tender) sites that overlie nerves and are not bony or hairy. The distance between the electrodes is chosen related to the intensity of the current — decreasing the distance increases its intensity because the current travels more superficially. With interferential stimulation, the currents need to cross in the targeted area (Kosses, 2004). Experiment with location and distance between sites to see what works best for your survivor.

How fast is pain relief? How long does it last?
With the proper site selection and adjustment to the unit, pain relief can be felt within ten to thirty minutes, using either the interferential or TENS units (Mannheimer, 1980). Relief can be felt within ten minutes using the TENS unit that doesn't produce a muscular contraction. Using the TENS setting that produces a muscular contraction, pain relief takes longer to achieve but it also lasts longer — more than an hour (Kosses, 2004). Pain relief from interferential units usually lasts longer (more than an hour) than with TENS units, although this depends upon the settings, duration of treatment, and unit used.

Who benefits and who doesn't from electrical stimulation units?
Those who use it to supplement their participation in clinical rehabilitation of an acute injury receive the greatest benefit. Thereafter,

it's a good first choice for pain relief after any kind of injury. Since your survivor is in control, he can also use it whenever he feels a need, post-rehab, and before a slight strain becomes a serious injury.

Although those with a complex pain syndrome who require pain medication may need more than an electrical stimulation unit, it can be part of a chronic pain management program.

What does research say about the electrical stimulation units?

As a choice for non-medication pain relief, they're very effective. Different theories explain why they work. An oft-repeated theory is that the electrical stimulation releases endorphins. Another explanation is that with injury, specific points related to the source of pain may be tender to the touch, feel fibrous, or show lower skin resistance than other neighboring areas, so stimulating these points reduces pain.

Additionally, scientists found that one or more acupuncture points were situated along the various peripheral nerves and overlying sensory end organs, suggesting the same anatomical structure is involved (Mannheimer, 1980). *Regardless of theory, they work!*

Orthotics and Foot Dysfunction

Spatial orientation: how it affects your survivor — and you.

Close your eyes and touch your nose with your right hand. How does your hand know where your nose is? For that matter, how does your brain know where your hand is? This complex sequence of events demonstrates how the brain gathers information from nerves throughout the body — without the use of your eyes. This process occurs all day long without our realizing it.

Did you know that basic foot dysfunction is one of the most common structural causes of neurological disorganization? This research finding is important for you and your survivor because when his proprioceptors (sensors that detect position in space) misread messages, more neurological stress is added to an already overloaded system (Rich, 1997).

Feet Sensors

The proprioceptors in your feet help you balance. As one of the most important sensors of your body's location in space, these nerves send information to the brain to organize muscles throughout the body.

For example, as you walk, stimulation of muscles, joints, and skin receptors in the foot provides information to your brain and then to the rest of your body to inform it which muscles to contract and which to relax to balance your posture and gait. When you stand, receptors in the feet are stimulated, and the postural extension muscles that keep you upright contract.

If your survivor's sensor system does not function properly due to abnormal motion within the foot, slumping replaces proper posture. His rounded shoulders, curved upper back, and lower swayback all occur because his postural extension muscles are not getting the proper information from his foot to contract!

The amazing foot and how we can achieve balance.

The feet, an amazing working system, contain over 25% of all the bones in our bodies. Twenty-six bones in each foot track and move together to allow us to walk properly. As we walk, our feet absorb one to three times our body weight. And, if you jump, this number goes up to five to seven times! (Rich, 1997).

Our daily activities and movement require equilibrium from a body that is not perfectly designed by nature. The most important imbalance comes from the fact that almost no one's legs are exactly the same length. The difference in leg length creates a less than ideal alignment of the feet.

Problems. The result of this imbalance? You name it, from tip to toe: head, neck, low-mid-upper back problems; hip, knee, calf, ankle, and foot problems. Why? Abnormally positioned feet do not allow physical stress to travel vertically from the feet toward the hip socket. Instead, the arches — which are not ideal anyway — allow physical vibrations to be transmitted diagonally toward the inner knee and low back region with every step taken. We may take about 6000-15,000 steps per day. Where is this unequal weight distribution felt? In most people these early signs of imbalance occur on the longer leg side of the body because there is more weight on that side.

Solutions. An evaluation by a professional who specializes in gait, alignment, and foot analysis is required to determine if your survivor — or you! — need corrective care. Foot dysfunction specialists may work in the fields of chiropractics, podiatry, orthopedics, rehabilitation medicine (physiatry), or physical therapy.

The first objective is to identify and correct the short leg with upper cervical adjustments; then achieve optimal foot alignment with custom-made orthotics. These shoe inserts minimize biomechanical faults, reduce joint wear and tear, and allow us to maximize performance — functional or athletic.

Personal experience. For several years I wore orthotics to correct leg-length differences, align my feet, and to provide arch support. My last model provided only a slight correction, so I gradually discontinued use. Now, as an aging athlete, I again require several pairs of orthotics to fit shoes for running, cycling, and dress. As important as balance is to performance — and thus to my sanity! — the investment is worth it. Try it and see!

Government Medical Insurance Programs

Medicare: Hospital and Medical Insurance

If your survivor receives Social Security Disability Income (SSDI), after a 24-month waiting period he automatically becomes eligible for Medicare. If he returns to work, he's covered through the trial work period and for 93 months beyond — if he's still considered disabled.

Medicare is divided into Part A, hospital; Part B, outpatient care (includes doctor visits, lab, and medical supplies); and Part D, drugs. Part A is premium-free. Part B requires either a willing doctor or joining an HMO. Part D requires you to select a drug plan, a Medicare Advantage Plan, or other Medicare Health Plan that offers drug coverage. Since Medicare and Social Security are hot national topics. Medicare coverage may change at any time.

Locating providers. To find providers who accept Medicare insurance, call Medicare customer service (800-633-4227) for a list or search the yellow pages and call to ask each doctor's billing staff. Either way takes time.

Payment for services. Medical professionals who agree to treat patients with Medicare insurance receive roughly 50% of the prevailing charge for services. To recover more of the charged amount requires payment by a supplemental insurance provider, such as Medicaid, Blue Cross, or an HMO. If you are eligible for both Medicare and Medicaid, the provider must accept both. Some providers just write off the remainder of the fee. Thank them if they accept Medicare payments because that means you won't be asked to pay any additional money.

Prescription drug coverage. The recent change in Medicare is complicated. You can join a prescription drug plan, a Medicare Advantage Plan such as an HMO or PPO, or another Medicare Health Plan that offers medication coverage. Before you choose, do Internet research or work with a local agency because once you choose, it's difficult to switch! The American Association for Retired Persons (AARP) is a source for current information on these plans (www.aarp.org).

If your survivor is low-income. If he's covered by Medicaid, he qualifies for "extra help" from any of the prescription medication plans. Be careful when selecting a plan to be sure that the co-pay is affordable. Almost all medication costs are covered but some medications require a minimal (usually $3 to $5) co-pay. Ask your physician to write prescriptions for a three-month supply so you can pay less often.

How much does Medicare pay for if he remains employed?
Currently, if he works and earns less than the Substantial Gainful Activity (SGA) limit, which was $970 in 2009, he'll continue to receive full coverage. He will pay premiums only if his income is above state limits for free coverage. If he earns more than the SGA and wants to keep Medicare coverage, he must pay a portion of his Part B premium ($96.40 per month in 2009). If his past earnings qualify, he may be eligible for reduced premiums. Those with employer-paid health plans may choose to purchase hospital insurance (Part A) separately. States will

pay hospital and medication coverage premiums for those with limited incomes. To learn if he qualifies, seek information from your local county health services agency, your state department of health and family services, or online from Social Security (www.ssa.gov).

Supplemental Medical Insurance: Medicaid

Low-income survivors are also eligible for supplemental insurance that can help pay for the Medicare prescription medication benefit, medical services, and necessities, such as eyeglasses. Those who work may receive continued coverage until their income reaches a certain level, which varies between states. If health care costs exceed the required income level, Medicaid continues as long as the disabling condition continues, your survivor needs coverage to work, and he's not able to afford similar health care coverage. Confused? Contact Medicare and your state Medicaid agencies to ask questions and to get the most current information about each system.

Locating Medicaid providers. To find health care professionals who will treat those of us on Medicaid insurance requires resourcefulness and perseverance. Why? Because the payment rate is low and the paperwork load is high. Some providers will accept Medicare-Medicaid — just ask. Some hospitals and all county clinics are required to accept Medicaid.

Personal experience. The best resources to locate medical assistance are your local brain injury association, rehab providers, and rehab/caregiver resource centers. Ask your survivor's team for referrals to their colleagues.

How to advocate for your survivor with a new doctor.
See also *Brain Injury Rewiring for Survivors.*

Do's:
   Before the appointment:
* Do research on expected treatment — consult others and Internet sources.

- Request time for questions and select a time of day when your survivor feels his best or worst, depending on what's needed.
- Make multiple copies of health history for the doctor and for you.

On the day of the appointment:
- Remind your survivor to eat — unless directed not to. Bring water and food if he can't eat before the appointment.
- Review questions and directions.
- Gather materials and bring copies for the doctor.
- Remind your survivor to discuss only the relevant issues.

At the appointment:
- Inform the provider that you and your survivor want to be fully informed of diagnosis, prognosis, treatment options/results, etc.
- Discuss contingency plans and follow-up appointments.

After the appointment:
- Help your survivor act upon treatment recommendations.
- Note any changes and ask your survivor what he notices.

If the desired response doesn't occur:
- Continue treatment as directed until the problem is resolved.
- Contact the doctor or designated person to discuss the problems.

Don'ts:
- Don't go to the appointment unprepared.
- Don't act or talk like a victim: "Look what they did/didn't do."

Some thoughts about doctors and our relationship with them.

Doctors may work for us, but their pay reflects more than money. Most doctors sweated blood and guts before, during, and after medical school, and they want to serve others. And, in this time of managed care, health professionals must do more with less. So, it is even more important to prepare for your visit and show respect.

> If you trust Google more than your doctor, then maybe it's time to switch doctors.
> — Jadelr and Cristina Cordova

Today, most doctors team with their patients for the best possible outcome. However, there may still be a few remaining old-school "retrogrouches" who believe that their MD equals "major deity"! If your doctor is one of these, change doctors!

Summary

Here are the points to remember about conventional medical intervention:

- Brain injury disrupts your survivor's brain and bodily functions.
- The body yearns to return to normal.
- To recover, your survivor must regain as much function as possible.
- To do that, his body needs to heal itself.
- For that to occur, self-trust is essential.
- Regardless of intent, too much intervention can confuse instinctual self-trust feelings and limit healing, rather than promoting it.
- Your survivor needs to be empowered to heal himself!

I know that my other most beloved therapist, the late Dr. Dale Johnson (DJ), would be quite pleased with himself and proud of me. I know you're in Heaven somewhere, DJ, chuckling at the can of worms you liberated on the earth!

Here are some thoughts about the best ways to help your survivor:

- Know the warning signs of depression.
- Effective medications are available. Discuss this with your doctor.
- Maintain social connections to reduce your own depression.
- Continue treatment with a therapist only if your survivor and the therapist like each other.
- Consider using EMDR and neurofeedback in his recovery.
- Explore using vision and balance therapy.
- Investigate new techniques to regain use of a damaged limb.
- Find aquatic, hippotherapy, and animal-assisted therapy programs.
- Seek expressive arts (music, drama, art) therapy programs.
- Consider using personal therapeutic devices such as a light box, etc.
- Investigate orthotics to correct structural misalignments.
- Prepare your survivor and his paperwork for medical appointments.

8

Mind, Body, Spirit Rewiring: Healing with Complementary Therapy

There are many paths up the mountain.
— Rabbi Marc Gellman

Ever since your survivor's injury, you've likely met innumerable conventional medical professionals — who practiced every conceivable brand of medicine — as you sought help for him to recover. You may feel discouraged about both his prognosis and his results so far and wonder if different treatments might work better. You're willing to try just about anything, even those unfamiliar to you. Good decision! This chapter will look at acupuncture, herbs, manipulation, massage, magnets, meditation, and other possibilities.

Introduction

Just as there are many paths when selecting a spiritual journey, there are a variety of ways to obtain and maintain health. People from different cultures carved paths that worked where they lived, and as a result several alternative forms of medicine developed. These systems continue to be practiced today as travelers successfully walk the same path to well-being that their ancestors took.

In this review of therapies that are complementary to traditional Western medicine, similarities among medical systems allow us to group them. Numerous ways for your survivor to heal, primarily from the Eastern perspective, will be presented. Some of these treatments and methods may seem peculiar. Certainly some will be mysterious. Others are likely to be questioned by those who are not up to date on the latest research and do not follow National Institutes of Health (NIH) recommendations. Still others may not be explored at all, not because they are not worthy, but because of time, energy, and experience limitations.

Treatments presented in this chapter are those I've experienced or that are closely allied with my recovery journey. I included a few of them because others strongly recommended their inclusion. We discuss:

- Holistic medicine.
- Traditional Chinese medicine: acupuncture, acupressure, and herbs.
- Aural energy healing: Qigong, Reiki.
- Physical energy healing: Jin Shin Jyutsu, Three Heart Balancing.
- Massage therapy: Shiatsu, reflexology.
- Other holistic medical treatments: naturopathy, osteopathy, homeopathy.
- Spinal manipulation.
- Other manipulative/chiropractic techniques: craniosacral, Network, BEST, Activator, Rolfing.
- Relaxation therapies: aromatherapy and hypnosis.
- Self-help therapies: magnets, imagery, meditation.

Holistic Medicine

The whole person is treated in this comprehensive system of care for our physical, emotional, social, spiritual, and economic needs. These principles are embraced (Bezilla, 1998):

- Each organism is greater than the sum of its parts.
- Every organism possesses an energy called *Chi, Qi,* Vital Force, or Spirit that lives throughout the system and must flow freely.
- Regularly consuming and enjoying air, animals, plants, sunshine, and water in their pure forms is necessary.

- Regular weight-bearing physical activity and repetitive dynamic movement is essential, like weight training, walking.
- A positive mental outlook includes stress management skills.
- Prevention of disease is superior to treatment of disease.

We start with traditional Chinese medicine (TCM), the oldest recorded holistic medicine, dating back to 1000 BC.

What is the Chinese medicine system and how do we know it works?
More than acupuncture, TCM is a complex medical system that has steadily evolved over the centuries. Practitioners first treat with acupuncture using one of its various traditions, then offer herbs and perhaps massage. They may recommend other compatible self-help modalities, such as acupressure, meditation, Qigong, and exercise, to assist their patients to achieve a balanced lifestyle of mind-body harmony.

How do we know that traditional Chinese medicine works?
The Chinese have used it to maintain health for thousands of years — even as early as the late Stone Age. Today, acupuncture is the treatment of choice for 500 million Chinese people, where success rates of 80-90% are reported (MacDorman, 1996), as well as millions of others throughout the world. *Would they use it if it weren't effective?*

According to Western medicine, if the treatment works, the hypothesis is correct and a theory is developed. This is basically how the TCM system and the elaborate *meridian* charts evolved over the centuries: noting the acupuncture points used to treat various conditions, and which organs corresponded with them (Tsuei, 1996).

What do conventional medical studies say?
TCM works! Impressed with the success of Chinese medicine, particularly the reduction of pain and nausea in certain circumstances, Western scientists used the scientific method to investigate, and reported results in respected medical journals (Rosenfeld, 1998).

In the fall of 1997, an independent panel at the U.S. National Institutes of Health (NIH) confirmed that acupuncture clearly works for several conditions and recommended integrating it into standard medical practice. The World Health Organization endorses its use for 40 ailments. One study of 10,000 Americans who were treated with acupuncture reported that 80% of them experienced significant improvement in their conditions (MacDorman, 1996).

Although Western scientists have yet to be able to identify either the bioelectrical energy flow system or any points along its path (because they cannot be seen), studies document that the brain releases natural painkillers when designated acupuncture sites are needled. (When needles are applied to a random site on the body not identified as an acupuncture point, symptoms are not relieved.) To further dispel placebo-effect doubters, advocates point to the success of acupuncture treatment, especially as an anesthetic, for animals (Tsuei, 1996).

> I'm less concerned about how it works than that it does. I think that qi, yin and yang, flow, and meridians express what's happening in the body in ways that we don't yet understand.
> — Major Steven Braverman

Origin of Traditional Chinese Medicine

Treating medical conditions with acupuncture needles can be dated back to the Sheng Dynasty in 1000 BC (Williams, 1996). Evidence inscribed on bones from this time documents both observations of medical conditions and their treatment with needles. It is believed that many Shamanic practices form the foundation of Chinese medicine. This spiritual link is clear — physical health and moral/spiritual life are inseparable.

Development of Energy Medicine in the West

Although the energy-system medical model was more developed in the East (particularly India and China), the idea of bioenergetic medicine was not new to Western medical investigators. In fact, 17th century scientists Galvani, Hahnemann, and Mesmer developed *vitalism*.

But acceptance of the concept waned in the 19th and 20th centuries, largely because Western medicine attempted to explain the energy system in orthodox medical terms. Also, technology was not advanced enough to measure the body's energetic processes, and thus a testable medical model could not be developed. A lack of financial support for scientific studies of acupuncture further delayed its acceptance.

Fortunately, 21st-century advances in physics, electro-magnetism, and other fields resulted in the first successful explanation of energy medicine. Today the Western version of the Chinese meridian theory uses modern terms to label and explain the traditional processes. For example, *chi* is called body energy and *meridians* are called pathways.

The theory behind bioenergy medicine is that energetic processes — electrical, magnetic, vibrational resonance, and biophoton emission — are crucial to all processes of life (Tsuei, 1996).

Traditional Chinese Medicine and Meridian Theory

Traditional Chinese medicine is based on the Taoist understanding that everything in the world is interdependent, interactive, and balanced. The same life force, called *chi* or *qi* (pronounced "chee"), is expressed differently by body, mind, and spirit and is a balance of the two complementary life forces, *yin* and *yang*, that are at work in all things in the physical and spiritual universe. If *yin* and *yang* are out of balance, disease results and doctors search for hidden forces that cause the disharmony. The goal is to recover balance (Williams, 1996).

Bodily energy, *chi,* generated by internal organs and systems, combines with breath to flow like a river and circulate throughout the body. In channels of high-density energy that vary from shallow to deep (1/16 inch to 1½ inches), fast to slow, weak to strong, the *chi* forms and travels along a complex, multi-layered system of paths called *meridians* that connect the various areas of the body, from internal to surface and back. This coordinated network of *meridians* directs the flow of *chi* throughout the body and controls all bodily functions (Williams, 1996).

These electrical energy *meridians* cannot be seen nor do they coincide with documented physiologic structures like nerves or arteries. But thousands of years of successful application validate that they exist.

Located along the 12 primary interconnected *meridians* on each side of the body, like ports on a river, are access points, called *acupuncture* points. *Chi* surfaces at these 360 sensitive spots on each channel. Energy can be drawn in or out of these points of high concentrations of *chi* flow, which are like miniature whirlpools or eddies in a river (Williams, 1996).

When the flow of *chi* is interrupted, health is disrupted, because *chi* sustains every life-giving function in the body. When there is an imbalance of the complementary life forces, the flow of energy is blocked. Pain, stagnation, and weakness result and lead to "dis-ease."

How does acupuncture work and what conditions does it treat?
It manipulates the flow of our bioenergy through the pathways in our bodies. Western science learned from experiments conducted over 200 years ago that the nervous system and the muscles operate with signals from tiny electrical charges that travel along nerve and muscle fibers. Recent research also suggests that the immune system and every biological system in the human body are influenced by the bioelectricity that travels in our fluids (MacDorman, 1992).

Endorphins and enkephalins, the body's natural pain-relievers, are released, as well as anti-inflammatory agents, growth hormones, and increased numbers of red and white blood cells — all inhibiting pain and speeding healing. Acupuncture balances hormones, blood pressure/flow, and the nervous system. Neurotransmitters, especially serotonin, are released, leading to feelings of calmness and serenity that promote emotional, mental, and physical healing (MacDorman, 1996).

In China, acupuncture has been used to treat every form of medical condition. In the West, while acceptance has been slow, the number of accepted applications is growing, most notably since the 1972 experience of *The New York Times* columnist James Reston who underwent an emergency appendectomy while traveling in China (Tsuei, 1996).

Best-known for pain relief, acupuncture is also effective on various biological systems, facial paralysis, and in treating nausea, vomiting, digestion problems, fibromyalgia (muscle and tendon pain), tinnitus (ringing in the ears), bronchitis, and asthma (Rosenfeld, 1998).

Additionally, ear acupuncture can be used for any condition, because all of the structures and organs of the body are represented on the ear. It is especially effective with acute pain of any type (Lewith, 1998).

How can acupuncture help survivors of brain injury?
Besides relieving the headache pain that often accompanies brain injury, acupuncture can also alleviate other chronic pain due to any cause, soft tissue injuries, and the addictions to drugs, alcohol, and tobacco that are common among survivors. Impaired immune systems and hormonal imbalances can also be corrected (Davids, 1997).

Acupuncture's effectiveness on various biological systems, including the digestive tract, cardiovascular, immune, and endocrine systems, is of special value because of our bodily disharmony (Tsuei, 1996). Successful treatment has also been demonstrated for a variety of brain injury-related conditions including hemiparalysis (paralysis of one side of the body), facial paralysis, degenerative arthritis of the cervical vertebrae, lumbago (pain in the lower back area), and herpes zoster (viral infection of spinal or cranial nerves).

Importantly, depression responds to acupuncture! Those who were needled at specific points were symptom-free after an eight-week study and even those treated at unrelated points improved (Davids, 1997)!

Addictions respond well to acupuncture and many drug addiction treatment clinics now use it. One center that combines acupuncture, counseling, and vocational and educational training reported that 75% of its graduates remained drug-free for two years (the length of the study), compared to 15-20% of standard clinic graduates (MacDorman, 1996).

Scalp acupuncture, a technique used in China since 1971, combines Western knowledge of neurological function and new needling techniques. Developed to treat brain injury survivors, scalp acupuncture can be started up to two years after onset or injury with beneficial results.

Reports demonstrate remarkable success: if treatment was begun immediately at the time of a stroke and then continued several times a week, few instances of post-stroke paralysis occurred if at least 50% of the nerve pathways were intact. Other injuries to soft tissue (nerves, muscles, tendons) that are usually slow to improve, healed at least 50% faster when treatment was begun immediately. Just like all types of acupuncture, response time for scalp acupuncture varies from immediate to delayed (MacDorman, 1996).

How many treatments are needed?

The number of treatments depends on how readily someone responds to acupuncture and how entrenched the condition is. For chronic conditions, a series of treatments spread over several weeks or months is necessary. Most practitioners suggest three to five treatments to assess effectiveness. Regular treatments are recommended at the change of seasons to help the body adapt to variations in climate.

How much do treatments cost? How do I find a practitioner?

Standard treatments with a licensed acupuncturist or MD usually cost $50-$100, depending on location. In 1997 the NIH recommended that medical providers include acupuncture as a treatment option and also urged insurance carriers to pay for acupuncture treatments. If a licensed doctor prescribes acupuncture for a specific purpose in the treatment of a properly diagnosed disorder, it is increasingly likely to be covered by insurance.

To find a practitioner, ask your health care team, satisfied patients, or a local acupuncture school. If results are not achieved after about five treatments, find someone else — there are many different traditions and treatment styles. Something will work!

Energy Healing

Practiced in many cultures, energy healing originates from a universal force that radiates from life itself. Energy healers "lay on hands" to move and redirect blocked energy. Many feel a connection

> The physician is only nature's assistant.
> — Galen

with the divine as they work to produce physical changes (Williams, 1996; Caldecott, 1996).

Although the various healing methods appear alike in their use of the human energy field, they differ in theory, approach, and application. Techniques are typically grouped into three basic categories, whether ancient or modern: healing of the aura, hands-on healing, and massage.

Healing of the Aura

Deriving from the Greek and Latin words for air, an aura is an energy field that surrounds the physical body about six inches away. We'll explore various methods that seek to redirect a person's energy.

Qigong

Using energy developed by practicing Qigong exercises, a therapist focuses her *qi* through a client's key acupuncture points to rebalance vital energy and to regain harmony. Although a growing body of evidence from China demonstrates that this energy healing practice works, many people, particularly in the West, remain skeptical. Certainly, because of the powerful energetic forces involved, it is vital to choose a practitioner who is thoroughly schooled and experienced in the theory and techniques (Williams, 1996).

Reiki

In this Japanese method, *Rei* is the God-consciousness and *Ki* is the universal life force. *Reiki* (pronounced "ray-kee") practitioners may place their hands on or above the body as their energy flows into the client through a series of positions. Perhaps because many *Reiki* masters are registered nurses, *Reiki*, like *Qigong*, is gaining the respect of the mainstream medical community. Many hospitals include some kind of *Reiki* program (Int'l Ctr. for Reiki Training, 2004; Mahoney, 2004).

Hands-on Healing

Although Western hands-on healers call their techniques many different names, these therapies all seem to be derivatives of the Japanese practice called *Reiki* described previously. Principles of all healing modalities include "Healing is teamwork. We healed you, not I healed you." Every act of healing is an act of prayer. "When love goes in, emotions flow freely" (Gardner, 2000).

Even though they are the recipients, clients are considered equal partners in the healing process, incorporating changes in diet, exercise, and self-awareness into their lifestyles.

Jin Shin Jyutsu

An ancient Japanese art of harmonizing the body's life energy, Jin Shin fell into relative obscurity until it was revived in the early 1900s and brought to the United States by Mary Burmeister in the 1950s.

As in TCM, Jin Shin Jyutsu adherents believe that a blocked energy pathway results in stagnation and can disrupt the local area, eventually disharmonizing the whole path of energy flow (JSJ, 2004).

Three Heart Balancing

The originator of this approach is Jaentra Green Gardener, who was diagnosed with multiple sclerosis and searched for 22 years to find any method that might help her overcome her illness. Seeking also to help others heal themselves, Gardner incorporated her many years of learning into this method, which focuses on the teamwork of healer, recipient, and God.

Although three hearts could refer to the preceding three partners, to Gardner, "Three Hearts" refers to the balance in the gravitational field in our bodies of what is called our third eye (located in the middle of the forehead), our physical heart, and our seat of *chi* (just below the navel).

How do I find hands-on healers?

Search the most common international names — Reiki, Healing Touch, Quantum Touch — that have well-developed training and credentialing programs. Another technique is called Polarity Therapy, which also incorporates cleansing diets and yoga-type exercises.

Massage Therapy

"Ahhh — this feels so good!" is a typical response from anyone who's experienced the soothing pleasures of massage. We know it's a potent stress reliever, but why does it feel so good? Massage stimulates the brain to produce endorphins, naturally controlling pain. Does it promote health to other systems beyond relaxation? Yes, massage is a healing art on all three levels — physical, mental, and spiritual.

What are the different kinds of massage?
Besides Swedish, there are many kinds that include acupressure, deep-tissue massage in which therapists use slow deep strokes to release chronic muscular tension, healing massage in which the healer works on the physical body and the aura in a warm quiet room with flowers or plants present (this technique is also more intense than conventional massage), Trager (a system of bodywork that uses gentle rocking and rolling of the client to loosen neuromuscular patterns that are inhibiting free movement), Zero Balancing (which involves both massage and gentle movement), Shiatsu, and reflexology.

Shiatsu
This pressure-point massage is similar to acupressure and can be used like a barometer of health. Practitioners diagnose and treat, according to what their sensitive hands determine as abnormalities in skin, body temperature, or muscles. Shiatsu utilizes the structures established by Western science to determine the location of points, which are linear and follow the skeletal and muscular form (Namikoshi, 1981).

Reflexology
Working on the hands and feet has been practiced throughout the ages by the Orientals and Egyptians. First developed in the early 1900s as Zone Therapy, reflexology holds with the theory that the body is comprised of ten zones, five on each side, corresponding to each toe and finger. More subtle than the observable system of nerves, reflexes travel through the zones from head to toe longitudinally, like electrical wiring. It is believed that excessive pressure on nerve endings from weakened muscle tissue in the feet results in congested blood flow, collection of waste products in the feet, and the formation of deposits. In a reflexology treatment, the feet are thoroughly massaged to break down these deposits (Horton, 1998).

What's the history of massage? Who says it works?
Massage is an ancient healing art. To Hippocrates, rubbing was one of the essential tools of physicians. Still practiced widely in Europe and Asia, back rubs were also part of standard nursing care in North America

until the early 20th century when modern medicine changed to treat exclusively with technology and medication (Moline, 1998)

Today a resurgence of interest in healing touch — Americans alone spend billions annually on massages — has spurred the medical community to investigate just how it helps. Massage treatments for patients with AIDS resulted in lower levels of stress hormones and more natural killer cells in the study participants in the massage group. These findings — that massage reduces stress and improves the immune system — led to research grants funded by the US National Institutes of Health to study medicinal massage (Moline, 1998).

Because of its traditional use to relax muscles and improve circulation, researchers speculated that massage would speed wound healing. It does! Measuring levels of stress hormones and blood pressure as indicators of healing, scientists found lower levels in the group of post-surgery patients who received a 45-minute massage for five days (Davids, 1997).

One study by a neurologist found that the physical touch of Swedish massage and acupressure helped 86% of those who did not respond to traditional pain treatment (medication, physical therapy, and ultrasound). Used as a treatment for insomnia, massage is also effective at reducing anxiety and increasing the ability to cope with hospital stress (Moline, 1998).

Personal experience. I'm one who doesn't need research studies to prove the benefits of massage. If I could afford it, I'd get a weekly rub! As an aging athlete who doesn't know when "enough is enough" until it's too much, therapeutic touch has replaced pain pills. I still demand a lot from my body and, because my injuries continue to tax my burdened system, my body yearns for bodywork just to participate in activities of daily life. In other words, I'm a walking advertisement for the benefits of massage! At one point I was lucky enough to barter my services (selling his used sports equipment) with a kind friend who enjoyed performing deep-tissue massage on other athletes so we could perform better. It was even better that he happened to be a chiropractor-athlete...

Other Holistic Medical Treatments

Naturopathy

Naturopathy is the heir to vitalism, the Western world's earliest entry into energy medicine. It embraces a belief in the vital force and natural healing powers of each person. As a holistic medical model, one treatment principle is that prevention is the best cure. It encompasses several practices: Oriental medicine, homeopathy, botanical medicine, manipulation, and other therapy modalities like electrical pulses (Naturopathic Medicine Network, 1998).

Homeopathy

"Let like be cured by like" is the treatise of this form of holistic medicine developed by German physicist and chemist Samuel Hahnemann in the late 1700s. Homeopathy employs the Hippocratic principle of "similars" — minute doses of natural substances that would elicit symptoms of illness in a healthy person are used to treat people with "dis-ease" from various conditions and illnesses. Chronic symptoms often respond best to homeopathy remedies. Conventional medicine employs the opposite principle to combat disease — strong doses are used to provide the contrasting reaction (Dannheisser & Edwards, 1998).

Although a staple of medical care in many countries of the world, homeopathy's growing popularity has mostly occurred in the last thirty years, especially in the US.

How might survivors benefit from homeopathy?

From a general standpoint, the holistic approach may benefit survivors. Homeopaths view a hierarchy of symptoms starting with the mental and emotional as they seek the cause of the dis-ease, and they see symptoms as deriving from a disturbed or weak life force. This is the same life energy that governs biological activity in the Chinese and Ayurvedic (Indian) systems of medicine (Dannheisser & Edwards, 1998).

Osteopathy

A relatively recent (1874) system of medical and surgical care, osteopathic medicine is based on principles similar to those of Hippocrates 2000 years earlier. Recognized as a standard treatment method, osteopathy differs from the more traditional medicine practiced in the US in its theory that the body can self-regulate if structural integrity is maintained.

Underlying all treatment is the principle that form and function work together. Although manipulation is the chief mode of restoring functional and structural balance to an injured system, doctors of osteopathic medicine (DOs) also rely on conventional physical, medicinal, and surgical methods. Medical training of osteopaths leads to licensure, just like with MDs, and DOs practice in all branches of medicine, although the majority of them are primary-care physicians (Bezilla, 1997).

What can osteopathic medicine specifically offer to survivors?

Many survivors develop biomechanical dysfunction from their injuries. A technique originally developed by William Sutherland, DO, in 1899, and popularized by John Upledger, can help your survivor. Cranial sacral therapy, practiced by osteopathic physicians in addition to chiropractors, is a gentle, yet powerful system that is believed to work by restoring the normal cranial rhythm that was disturbed with injury or disease.

Cranial osteopathy, treating the whole body from the biomechanical perspective, is used to care for those with asthma and other ear-nose-throat problems, in addition to muscle tension headache, cerebral palsy, and other cranial-associated diseases and conditions (Feeley, 1998).

Spinal Manipulation/Chiropractic

Stories of curing paralysis by aligning neck vertebrae to restore nerve transmission are seen in ancient manuscripts (Rondberg, 1996). We're rediscovering it works for us, too! Following an extensive study of all available care for low back

> Get knowledge of the spine, for this is the requisite for many diseases.
> — Hippocrates

problems, the Agency for Health Care Policy and Research (AHCPR) recommended that spinal manipulation is the only safe, effective, medication-free form of initial professional treatment for acute low back problems in adults.

Ninety percent of Americans who used chiropractic care reported the treatments were effective and those with back problems were more satisfied with chiropractic treatment than any other type of care (ACA, 1998). Primarily recognized as an effective treatment for low back problems, chiropractic is covered by medical insurance carriers, although a limit on the number of visits per year or injury is often imposed.

How can chiropractic especially help survivors of TBI?

The many different areas of pain that resulted from your survivor's injury can be effectively treated with chiropractic care. Headache, as well as back, neck, and joint pain respond to the hands-on approach that restores joint mobility, thereby alleviating pain and muscle tightness, and allowing tissues to heal.

***Personal experience**: I'll never forget how I first learned about chiropractic. I was teaching half-time in the fall after my January car crash when a colleague started talking about how much better her neck felt after a chiropractic treatment — a whiplash-type injury two weeks earlier had already subsided!*

On the other hand, my neck injury that occurred nine months previously was still not better despite physical therapy, massage, traction, cortisone injections, Valium — the whole nine yards of conventional medical care. Hmm, I thought. This calls for further investigation — I wonder how long before my neck feels better? I think I'll give this chiropractor thing a try — can't hurt anymore than it does — and it might get better just like Marlys' did — without the side effects of medications!

I went to her doctor, felt better, and continue to seek chiropractic care wherever I live. Even if I feel okay, I always feel better when my head is screwed on right. Just day-to-day living, sleeping, driving, sports, or tension can cause misalignment of the cervical vertebrae after they've been injured. I lift weights to strengthen the supporting musculature so the adjustment holds better, and now I'm a believer, too!

Other Manipulative Techniques

Besides spinal manipulation, other specialized kinds of treatment performed by chiropractors — and osteopaths, naturopaths, massage therapists, and others — can be a boon to your survivor, especially cervical and cranial-sacral therapy.

Those of us whose injuries include whiplash or contrecoup impact are good candidates for these treatments for our cervical and cranial-sacral system because the membrane that encases our brain probably developed unhealthy adhesions and tensions after the brain impacted the inside of the skull. Bones that have moved out of place hold the membrane in an abnormal, unnatural, and dysfunctional position until they are restored to their rightful place

Our cranial-sacral system, composed of the bones of our skull, face, and mouth, extends by a system of hydraulics and membranes to the lower end of the spine. An injury to any part of the system affects all of it — *where have we heard this before?* For example, even a minor fall on the tailbone affects the system all the way to the cranium, perhaps resulting in headache or irritability (Upledger, 1983).

Cranial-sacral therapy. After assessing the cranial-sacral system to detect imbalances and movement restrictions, a therapist uses gentle manual techniques to release problem areas and relieve excessive pressure on the brain and spinal cord. Essentially, the therapist removes the obstacles that the normally self-correcting physiological forces have not been able to dislodge and empowers the body to do the rest. When healthy, the body's inherent hydraulic system can be relied upon to contribute toward the maintenance of this corrective process. A session may last from 15 minutes to more than an hour; the initial evaluation may be enough to correct the problem (Upledger, 1983, 2001). Many conditions can improve or be alleviated with this treatment.

Personal experience. My best friend Marlys, who introduced me to the wonders of chiropractic in 1976, saw my vocabulary dramatically improve as a result of craniosacral treatments. Although I'd majored in English in college, she hadn't seen any evidence of advanced vocabulary after my injury until my treatments in the 1980s.

I thought I was more articulate, but you know how it is with us survivors — we're skeptical of any signs of progress because we wonder if it's real and how long it'll last. The return of my vocabulary is a good indication that cranial-sacral therapy works — removing obstacles permits the body to self-correct.

Network spinal analysis cues the nervous system to self-regulate by light touch applied to *spinal gateways*. And it's effective! Self-reports from 2818 patients indicated that 76% of them made statistically significant improvement in many wellness areas. These included physical and mental/emotional states, response to stress, improved life enjoyment, and overall quality of life during a one-year period of care. The longer people were in care, the greater the benefits! (Epstein, 2000).

BEST (Bio Energetic Synchronization Technique) is a mind/body healing method. BEST practitioners adhere to the principle of mind-body-spirit balance for optimal health. When any of these energy fields is out of balance, people develop symptoms and ill health follows. Because emotions and thoughts play such a big role in our health, the BEST approach utilizes a system of light touch on certain pressure points to restore the energy field as a client thinks about a specific memory stress. Adherents have found that the body can repair and rebuild following the procedure, especially when other causative factors are addressed, such as diet, exercise, sleep, cleanliness of air, and mental stress (Morter, 2002).

Personal experience. One of my treating chiropractors, Todd Binkley, uses both BEST and Network techniques on me. After seeing him for a year or so we both noticed that my default emotion of anger had been replaced! Now, it is more likely to be joy. It can also be anxiety or confusion, but everything beats anger! (I see him monthly to keep tuned).

Activator methods. These involve a low-force, high-speed adjustment technique for joint dysfunction in the spinal column and extremities. Using a spring-loaded device about 6" long with a rubberized tip the size of a fingernail, a chiropractor aims it at a misaligned bone and this activator instrument moves the bone right back in place! Evolved from over 35 years of empirical study and 15 years of clinical research, this technique is the most widely used technique worldwide with over 35,000 trained chiropractors. It is also preferred by those for whom the full force chiropractic adjustments are too powerful or for whom they aren't as effective (Activator Methods Int'l, 2004).

Personal experience. I love the activator! Because it's gentle and effective, my body now prefers this kind of adjustment. Chiropractor Olivia Herrell first used it on me a few years ago after another mountain biking fall and I still use it I because it works!

Rolfing/structural integration aims to re-align and harmonize the body to operate more easily and efficiently. Performed in a sequence of 10 sessions, practitioners of this technique use deep — and often painful — manipulation to loosen or release connective tissue (fascia) adhesions around the muscles that restrict movement. Beginning with the feet, Rolfers use a standardized system of physical manipulations that are designed to reeducate the body to a better way of moving. New gentler techniques are now used to create these changes without pain (Rolf Institute, 2004).

Personal experience. I wish those pain-free methods had been available when I was "Rolfed" in the early 1980s!

Two techniques that I've not experienced look effective: Neural Organization Technique (NOT) and Sacro-Occipital Technique (SOT).

NOT. Using digital pressure on acupuncture and other points as well as on the lymphatic system, this non-invasive technique is designed to correct bodily faults that disorganize the central nervous system (Ferreri, 2004).

SOT. It focuses on the relationship between the sacrum and the occiput. In this technique, the body is specifically positioned to use its weight to correct the cranial-sacral respiratory mechanism malfunction (SORSI, 2002). This may work well for whiplash and fall injuries.

Relaxation Therapies

Several other non-traditional therapies have helped me. Here are some of the most useful.

Aromatherapy

"Use fragrances to treat brain injury? You're kidding, right?"

Well, actually no. Healing with scented massage oils and incense has been practiced for at least 6000 years. Remember when the Three Wise Men brought gifts of frankincense, gold, and myrrh to celebrate the birth of Jesus? Egyptians valued these essences, which were traditionally offered to the sun and moon gods, and the Chinese burned incense to show respect to the gods. Traditional Indian medicine used healing aromas, as did South and North American Indians.

The word *aromatherapy* came from a French chemist who accidentally burned himself, immersed his hand in lavender oil, noted how quickly the burn healed, and published a book about the anti-microbial effects of the oils. Further research on the healing powers of oils led to the massage method of applying the oils to the skin — this form of aromatherapy is now used worldwide.

Reduction in stress and anxiety and improvement in sleep and sexual performance are reported. A brain injury survivor of carbon monoxide poisoning used essential oils, aromatherapy, and Chinese whole food concentrates in her recovery (Aroma Web, 1998).

Personal experience. As part of treatment, my former acupuncturist, Claudia, gently massaged tiny quantities of different oils into the soles of my feet following needle insertion to further relax and heal me. My friend Marlys treats me with essential oils during her energy work and I find they help heal my various muscle and tendon injuries.

Imagery Techniques

We all know how our minds can transport us somewhere else. Remarkable as it seems, the scenes we imagine actually influence involuntary bodily processes. Research on the various imagery approaches — guided imagery, hypnosis, meditation, and biofeedback — demonstrate this amazing ability of humans to self-regulate.

More than physiology is influenced, however. As a connection between body and mind, imagery can serve as a useful tool to understand causes of dis-ease. When the analytical part of the mind sorts through the new information and decides on a course of action, healing can occur.

Trained therapists can help survivors see how their thinking influences how they feel and how to use this tool to help themselves recover.

Guided imagery and how it helps survivors

Taking an imaginary journey under the direction of a chosen voice, either in person or on a recording, is what this technique is all about. Fully conscious participants venture to a pleasant place for a five to ten minute journey. Some choose to involve their senses as they feel, smell, hear, and taste their experience. Following the imaginary escape, several different activities may occur, depending on the setting.

If it's a counseling session, your survivor may explore a trip with a therapist. In a writing seminar, he may log it in a journal, then perhaps share his experience with others in the group, with or without psychological interpretation. Privately, he may write about his venture in a journal or talk into a tape recorder. If he's preparing for a medical procedure, he can rehearse a successful outcome, and picture everyone involved doing their part.

When stress plays a role in emotionally responsive ailments such as headache, neck and back pain, digestive disorders, heart palpitations, dizziness, fatigue, or anxiety, imagery techniques can help to relieve the emotional pain. Even major health problems like heart disease, cancer, and neurological illnesses that cause or are complicated by stress and anxiety are often helped by imagery (Rossman, 1998).

Hypnosis

Under the direction of a trained therapist, a sleep-like state is induced in a willing participant, who is then particularly susceptible to the suggestions of the hypnotist. Used to control pain, cope with painful memories, and control obsessive behavior, hypnosis can be a powerful therapeutic tool. People can also learn self-hypnosis techniques to manage various problems themselves. Although a hypnotic experience involves a reduced sense of awareness, a willing participant still controls his actions — we're just more open to ideas than in a fully conscious state.

Meditation

Meditation in all of its forms has been practiced for thousands of years for its spiritual and health benefits as it quiets minds and bodies.

Meditation decreases heart rate, respiratory rate, blood pressure, and oxygen consumption as it offers protection against anxiety and depression. Alpha waves — brain waves indicating a state of relaxed alertness which are rarely found during sleep — are plentiful during meditation. In a peaceful state, your survivor may more easily find solutions for problems.

Various studies show that those who meditate experienced reduced pain from muscle tension, headache, and other conditions. Healing one mode of consciousness — the mind — changes another mode — the body. Some studies also show enhanced functioning of the right hemisphere of the brain, which is associated with creativity and imagination (Redwood, 1998). See *Brain Injury Rewiring for Survivors* for specific techniques.

Magnetic Therapy

The idea of healing with magnets isn't new. Many different cultures throughout the ages have reported the medical use of magnets — and their results were questioned — until November 1997 when a rigorous test directed by two skeptical scientists demonstrated the powers of magnetic therapy or energy medicine, as it is sometimes called (Altman, 1997).

The Chinese believe that, like acupuncture, magnets restore our *chi* flow. Advocates suggest that there is a correlation between sensitivity to acupuncture and magnetic therapy — those most responsive to acupuncture will be the most responsive to magnets.

How can survivors be helped?
Many areas can be treated. Let's start with the head. Headache pain responds to a magnetic headband or to magnets taped on the temple area or the back of the head, just above the neck. Insomnia can be treated by placing a magnet on the forehead between the eyebrows for 10 minutes at bedtime. Better sleep is promised after a few days (Weil, 1998).

Back pain is relieved with a magnetic back brace, a strip magnet, or by taping magnets on both sides of the spine. Arthritis pain and repetitive stress injury respond to a magnetic band worn on the wrist or around the elbow or to magnets taped to the affected joints. Fibromyalgia and systemic arthritis pain may be treated with a magnetic mattress pad. For various types of foot pain and problems, magnetic insoles are often effective (Lawrence, 1998; Weil, 1998).

Personal experience. After reading the Lawrence article on magnet therapy, I decided to give it a try for a 12-week case of elbow tendonitis aggravated by continuous computer use. The pain prevented me from weeding and cleaning, which I didn't mind, but it also interfered with my sports activities, which I did mind!

As I charged into the magnet store, I remember the marked contrast between the peaceful appearance of the owner and my own sense of urgency and pain. The owner immediately asked me if I wanted to sit down on a magnetic cushion (hmm... I wonder why?).

I assured him I preferred to stand and started my onslaught of questions, surrounded as I was by magnets in a variety of belts, wraps, supports, cushions, pillows, and mattress pads. For my elbow and head pain, he handed me an expandable magnetic bracelet and a pair of magnetic earrings. Then I slipped on a necklace and a back belt, and sat on a magnetic cushion where I also tried on a magnetic mask. Instantly, my head ached. Oops! Too much magnetism, but I realized my elbow pain was gone. This got my attention! For my limited finances, sluggish brain, and movable pain needs, I settled on a pair of gold earrings and a pad of eight 900-Gauss magnets, powerful and portable enough to use anywhere. Utilizing one of my many wraps, I wore the pad on my elbow and the magnetic earrings as I worked on the computer with a refreshed brain for several days — still no pain. Then I challenged the elbow with a weight workout. The pain did not return and my brain worked better.

I also wore the pad on my chest (to strengthen lungs) and then moved it to my pillow to sleep on. Almost immediately, with the magnets on my pillow, my sleep quality improved so I needed less than my usual 10 hours. As I work to complete the book, I am thankful for the magnets.

Summary

As we know, "There are many paths up the mountain." I hope that you and your survivor explore some — or many — of these alternative ways of healing and incorporate them into your lives. Seek until you find what works for all of you. May God bless your journey.

- Prevention of disease is superior to treatment of disease.

> The physician is only nature's assistant.
> — Galen

- Every organism possesses an energy (called *chi, qi,* Vital Force, Spirit) that lives throughout the system and must flow freely.
- Acupuncture can correct imbalances and alleviate pain.
- Addictions and depression respond well to acupuncture.
- Investigate energy and hands-on healing methods.
- Know that many different kinds of massage are beneficial.
- Explore naturopathy, homeopathy, and osteopathy.
- Chiropractic care effectively treats back, neck, and joint injuries.
- Other manipulative techniques work, too.
- Imagery, hypnosis, meditation, and magnetic therapy can be beneficial.

9
Nutritional Rewiring: Healing with Healthy Eating and Lifestyle

> Food plus joy equals health.
> — National Nutrition Council of Norway

What your survivor puts into his body affects how he feels. No surprise there. What is surprising is that good nutrition is not that hard to achieve.

Introduction

Although eating and living healthfully is a personal choice, you can encourage, cajole, and help your survivor in this vital aspect of his rewiring. His nutritional chapter explains why he needs optimal nutrition and how he can obtain it. This chapter covers:

- How his injury impacted his body and how nutrition helps.
- How you can help your survivor to eat healthfully.
- How medications interact with food.
- Serving-size guide.
- Ways to reduce calories and add flavor to food.
- How supplements can help to heal him.

Here's to healthful living for all of you!

What brain injury conditions require nutritional intervention?

All neurological conditions need extra care. To understand the reasons, let's review some information found in our general rewiring chapter.

First, remember that your survivor's initial brain injury resulted in a massive biochemical cascade of reactions that traumatized his entire system. His wiring is a mess. Some wires were severed, some were pinched, some temporarily disconnected, and some were damaged beyond repair. Others may appear undamaged but cannot operate as they once did. And, when functioning neurons die, other nerve fibers compete for the vacant positions (Stein, 1995).

Second, all of the trauma to his cell tissue — the tearing, bleeding, swelling, and breakdown of cell membranes — led to the formation of substances called free radicals, the renegade chemicals that continue to create even more havoc, especially with weakened cells.

Not only does he need healthy food to recover, but his brain also is more susceptible to damage by these free radicals. Decades of research show that the initial trauma initiated a chronically progressive degenerative process and that the neurological trauma is aggravated by the presence of free radicals (Berker, 1996 and others).

Third, following treatment of acute symptoms, your survivor is at risk for several delayed complications — seizures, neurotic and psychotic disorders, increased suicide risk, reduced life expectancy, earlier onset of stroke and the changes of old age, progressive intellectual degeneration, and development of post-traumatic stress syndrome (PTSD) symptoms. Although this wide-ranging list is certainly depressing, research supports it (Berker, 1996; Faden, 1996).

Finally, to help you remain hopeful, remember that your survivor's brain attempts to rewire itself after his trauma. The reserve capacity of the brain for reorganization and recovery is cause for optimism. The brain recovers and repairs by regenerating, sprouting, compensating, and adapting. In this process, some wires substitute for injured ones, either temporarily or permanently, some sprout new growth to replace a damaged section, and other wires try to repair themselves. Fortunately, human ability to adapt to changes and still function is not dependent on the exact rewiring of damaged circuits.

Can nutrition repair damage? What kinds?

Yes. Any condition short of death can improve if vital nutrients are available. Although medication plays a more dominant role in correcting biochemical imbalances from the injury, diet influences the effectiveness of his medications, as well as his general body chemistry.

Studies found that treatment with antioxidants, specifically Vitamin E, slows disease progression caused by oxidative stress from free radicals and slows cognitive decline in older persons — his injury effectively gave him a brain older than his years. Both the intake of supplements and consumption of foods high in antioxidants, like fruits and vegetables, contribute to these improvements (Morris, et al., 2003; Gemma et al., 2002).

While his current lifestyle and nutritional plan cannot affect the initial impact/illness, he can arrest the "rusting" while research seeks medication and nutritional strategies to treat brain trauma and repair damaged cells.

How can I help my survivor to eat healthfully?

You know that your survivor's food and lifestyle choices can either heal him or hurt him. You also know that he controls what he eats and that old habits and tastes die hard. So, what can you do? To help him to eat healthfully and lead a lifestyle that helps him to rewire and recover:

- Discuss his nutritional chapter with him.
- Remind him that his "car" needs premium fuel to run well.
- Discuss with him how bad food choices slow his recovery.
- Buy and prepare healthy food and order it when you dine out.
- Help him find ways to treat any substance dependencies.
- Encourage him to create a routine for refreshing sleep.

Nutrition Questions and Answers

What counts as a serving?

Think of a reasonable amount to eat at one time. Typical servings are one medium piece of fruit, six ounces of juice, one to two cups of greens, one slice of bread, one cup of milk, two to three ounces of meat or fish (the size of a deck of cards), or one ounce of cereal (which varies in size; for example, one ounce of granola may be only ¼ cup but one ounce of a puffed rice or wheat cereal may be more than one cup). This table has a guide to serving sizes for some other foods:

Food	Official serving	Approx. size
Cheese	1 oz.	1" cube or 2 slices
Ice Cream	½ cup	a tennis ball
Meat, chicken, or fish	2-3 oz.	deck of cards
Beans	½ cup cooked	
Butters (almond, peanut, etc.)	1 oz.	2 Tablespoons
Pasta or rice	½ cup cooked	a tennis ball
Cooked vegetables	½ cup cooked	a tennis ball
Raw vegetables (Greens)	1 cup	big handful
Fresh fruit	1 medium-size, ½ cup, ½ grapefruit	
Dried fruit	¼ cup	a large egg

How can we eat enough servings of fruits/veggies and whole grains?
Enjoy several servings at every meal and snack on them. For example, breakfast could include a glass of juice, an egg, and a slice of whole-wheat toast with jam, or a banana with cereal and milk or yogurt.

Personal experience. When I jump out of bed I can't wait to eat my favorite breakfast of cereal, yogurt, and fruit, and a few cups of coffee! For a bottom layer, I enjoy a variety of whole grain cereals, choosing hot in winter and cold in summer. Next I spoon a mixture of non-fat vanilla and non-fat plain yogurt combined with in-season fruit. I top this with ground flaxseed for omega-3, soy granules, and walnuts. This morning meal is such a winner that it also makes a light supper, bedtime snack, or a special dessert — with chocolate added, of course! Yum!!

How do his medications interact with food and affect appetite?
Food and beverages may either intensify the effects of a drug or conflict with it. For example, dairy products interfere with the absorption of the antibiotic tetracycline, so that neither is absorbed. Other drugs, like aspirin, can upset an empty stomach. Caffeine reduces the sedating properties of antihistamines and some antidepressants and increases effects of pain-relievers. Supplements need food for the best nutrient

absorption, which is why we take them with meals. Alcohol intensifies the sedating properties of medications.

Medications may increase or decrease appetite. Some drugs that may increase appetite include many antidepressants, antihistamines (allergy pills), diuretics, and tranquilizers.

Foods and medications can each change the acidity in our digestive tracts and affect absorption — for better or worse. For example, acidic beverages, like colas and grapefruit juice, can interfere with antibiotics and other medications. Diuretics increase water loss and can eliminate essential electrolytes like potassium.

Drugs that may decrease appetite include antidepressants, antibiotics, and medications that treat seizures, high blood pressure, or high cholesterol. Some medications may even cause nausea — or worse — or reduce appetite, intentionally or not. Do you notice antidepressants are listed in both lists? This is because different drugs within a class of drugs affect each person's appetite differently. For example, Prozac (fluoxetine) may decrease or increase appetite, depending on the individual response. Because many different interactions can occur, observe what happens to your survivor and then confer with your health professionals. Pharmacists are a good source of information about medications.

Personal experience. Weight gain runs counter to all of my fitness goals as well as my self-image. When I experienced sleep problems after a long successful run with Prozac, my physician suggested I try a new medication. One possible side effect was increased appetite, which I experienced, so we stopped it immediately. I resumed taking Prozac with a different medication for sleep. It worked — and my appetite was under control again. I no longer take Prozac, but the lesson remains an important one. Keep experimenting until you find what works best for you!

Are carbohydrates good or bad to eat?
Carbohydrates (carbs) can be healthful (e.g., vegetables or fruit) or unhealthful (e.g., candy or soda). They are currently a hot news topic perhaps because Americans today are fatter than ever, despite years of focus on low-fat eating. Why? Former diet wisdom said that eating fatty

food caused cholesterol problems and diseased hearts. So people replaced slow-burning fats with fast-burning carbohydrates and chose "low-fat" foods, in which sugar replaced fat. What happened? Because they were hungrier (some fat is needed for a sense of fullness and satisfaction after a meal), people ate more food, especially if something was labeled low- or non-fat or cholesterol-free. Many didn't consider calories, since the mantra was "fat makes us fat!"

Tragically, the "fat phobic" message had little impact on heart disease. Instead, it led to an obesity epidemic, and more people developed sugar diabetes, insulin resistance, and metabolic syndrome. Help your survivor select healthy carbohydrates to avoid more illnesses and increased brain damage!

How shall we choose which carbohydrates to eat?
To make it simple, just fill your plates with vegetables! If you want to be informed, consult various charts, too. After a while, you'll remember which foods are high or low in sugar, as well as calorie and fat content.

If you like potatoes, the best choices are sweet potatoes, yams, and new potatoes. Serving baked potatoes with sour cream and butter adds lots of high-fat calories.

If you and your family enjoy bread, eat the whole grain variety, which provides more fiber and less added sugar. The package should feel heavy. Make sure that a whole grain (e.g., cracked wheat) is listed first on the ingredient list rather than refined flour and sugar.

Buy whole-grain pasta and tortillas, too. Cereals can contain lots of added sugars. Beware! Check lists of ingredients and buy the unsugared varieties containing oat and wheat.

If you like rice, buy brown, basmati, or (my favorite) jasmine rice rather than white rice. Most vegetables, including carrots, corn, and bean, are good choices. The same goes for fruit.

What are some ways to reduce calories and not sacrifice flavor?
Our taste buds learn to like what they taste the most. So, give them less saturated fat and sugar and watch the cravings disappear! Think of what you like about a particular food. Is it the texture? The taste? Then try these ideas:

- Try baked chips instead of fried — most are fried and there's a huge difference in fat.
- Remove the skin from poultry.
- Broil, microwave, bake, or grill instead of frying.
- Use cooking sprays instead of butter or margarine — or use one of those pressurized containers to which you can add your own oil.

> We are indeed much more than what we eat, but what we eat can nevertheless help us to be much more than we are.
> — Adelle Davis

- Try low-fat spreads, but check that they're transfat-free.
- Replace regular high fat and/or sugar products with reduced/non-fat or low-sugar ones. Then combine or try just the reduced versions and see if you still like them, like salad dressing, mayo, milk, yogurt, etc.
- Substitute plain non-fat yogurt for sour cream or combine them.
- Use dry or fresh fruit, salsas, and balsamic vinegar to pep-up bland foods or to replace fat for flavor. Try salsa on corn-on-the-cob!
- Experiment with spices.
- Try Stevia, an herbal no-calorie sweetener, instead of sugar.
- Dilute your favorite beverages with soda water.
- Choose an unsweetened beverage or water — but not "diet" beverages. Chemical sweeteners in them can actually make you hungrier.

How can we encourage him to eat more leafy greens?
Serve a variety and in combination. Try different low fat salad dressings and/or vinegar-oil or lemon juice-oil. Vinegar is available in different flavors to use with olive oil. Spray containers that save money and ensure only a small amount of oil is used can be found on-line or in stores. Combining vinegar with olive oil is also low-cost! For more interest, add sliced nuts, raisins, shredded veggies (like carrots) or green onions, and spices to basic greens. For variety, place a protein source, like fish, chicken, tofu, meat, or beans on a bed of greens, along with rice. To help warm your bodies in the winter, lightly steam greens (microwaving is easy) with sliced ginger and garlic. Invite him to join in food preparation — it can be fun and helps his recovery in several ways!

Are wilted greens a problem? Keeping greens fresh is no sweat when you place a paper towel in the bag of washed greens to absorb excess moisture. Special bags are also available to keep produce fresh.

How can we protect our family from pesticides on our produce?

Buy organic and/or spray the hard fruits and vegetables with a commercial or homemade vinegar-water combination. The vinegar kills bacteria and removes wax and most pesticides. To make your own: add two tablespoons of white vinegar to eight ounces of water in a spray bottle. Scrub with a vegetable brush. Rinse thoroughly with cool water.

What can we do about his lactose intolerance? Why is yogurt good?

Research suggests that gradually introducing small amounts of milk products into your diet may reduce the unpleasant side effects, if not erase the problem entirely. Or perhaps try soymilk, goat milk, or lactose-free milk. Another solution is to consume milk products like yogurt, buttermilk, or sour milk, which may be considered "predigested" because a bacteria has been added that digests the lactose.

Because yogurt coats the intestinal lining, it is often recommended if digestive problems arise from inadequate digestive enzymes. Additionally, those who undergo chemotherapy derive some benefit from the friendly bacteria in yogurt because cancer-killing drugs also kill the "good bacteria" that are needed for digestion.

What does research say about vitamin supplementation?

Early results look very promising for brain injury survivors! One study looked at how antioxidant therapy affected degenerative conditions, which are exacerbated by brain injury. Most of the conditions for which your survivor is at risk are degenerative.

Study participants in the early stages of Parkinson's disease and before medication treatment were given high doses of vitamin E and vitamin C (the exact amounts were not divulged in the study). The good news is that they did not need treatment with medication until 2½ years later than people who were not given these antioxidants.

This finding is important because, although the progression of Parkinson's disease was not stopped, the antioxidants kept the symptoms from progressing as fast to the stage that medication intervention was needed, thus providing a better quality of life for a longer period of time (Margen, 1992).

Other studies prompt scientists to strongly suggest that Vitamin E may combat the effects of traumatic brain damage better than they fight degenerative diseases, but either way, we're winners!

Supplements provide both psychological assurance and physical insurance that his antioxidant needs are met to neutralize the free radical damage from his injuries and daily living.

He likes beer and wine. Can he safely drink alcohol?
Check with your physician to determine how the effects of alcohol interact with his medications and then discuss quantity. Other ways to gain the heart-protective (blood-thinning) effects of alcohol are to drink grape juice and eat grapes, chocolate, and other foods that contain flavonoids, like garlic, onions, broccoli, and lemons. If it's the taste he enjoys, experiment with non-alcoholic beverages to find substitutes.

Remind him not to rely on alcohol to provide the neurochemicals that his brain needs; his medications are designed to do this. If he experiences a food or drink craving, investigate the cause. Has there been a change in eating, exercising, or sleeping patterns? Has his water intake decreased? Perhaps the dark days of winter increase his need for serotonin and he wants to eat more carbohydrates. Observe and discuss with your physician — rewiring is a dynamic process! And remember that there are other adverse effects of alcohol use! See Chapter 6 in *Brain Injury Rewiring for Survivors.*

Personal experience. I love the flavor of beer and wine, especially with meals! Trusting me to control my alcohol intake, my physician agreed that I could enjoy an alcoholic drink with food, which slows absorption. Adding sparkling water to the wine saves calories and alcohol! If I only want a taste of beer, I pour the rest on my rose bushes to repel various insects!

Summary

You know that your survivor's food and lifestyle choices can either heal him or hurt him. You also know that he controls what he eats and that old habits die hard. Because your survivor's mind and body no longer function as they once did, his former food habits don't work either.

> Hospitality consists in a little fire, a little food, and an immense quiet.
> — Ralph Waldo Emerson

What can you do? You can be good role models if you follow the suggestions in his chapter and provide the good food he needs. If you don't purchase junk food, he can't eat it! To help him to eat healthfully and lead a lifestyle to optimally rewire:

- Discuss his nutritional chapter with him.
- Remind him that his "car" needs premium fuel to run well.
- Discuss with him how bad food choices slow his recovery.
- Help him to choose healthy carbohydrates and eat more produce.
- Buy and prepare healthy food and order it when you dine out.
- Help him find ways to treat substance dependencies.
- Encourage him to create a routine for refreshing sleep.

10
Physical Rewiring:
Healing His Body with Exercise

> The only thing that ever sat its way to success was a hen.
>
> — Sarah Brown

Brain Injury Rewiring for Survivors strongly urges your survivor to get active and play to enjoy life and create new brain cells. Here we further explore the mental and physical benefits of exercise. Did you know that survivors who exercise far surpass those who don't? We discover why and how physical activity helps survivors to recover and look at typical physical problems and places that offer help. This chapter covers:

- Benefits of exercise, including recent research.
- Recovery process — typical problems and common deficits.
- Before he starts — preparation, goals, motivation.
- Helpful equipment.
- Programs to improve his movement.
- Accessible gardening.

Introduction

You will probably hear something like this from your survivor: "Yeah, right, physical recovery — I don't think so! Heal my injured body myself? It's not gonna happen. My body is so damaged there's nothing left to recover. It's hopeless. Nothing I can do will bring it back."

Encourage him to try. Encourage him to adapt the "Use it or lose it" motto and say, "Use it to lose it!" Lose what? How about his disability?

If he argues that nothing can take that away, you can say, "You're right. However, if you exercise, you'll be less disabled — isn't that better than the way things are now?"

There are several ways he can achieve this goal. Besides exercise, muscle-stimulating devices and Constraint-Induced therapy (see Chapter 7) also strengthen affected limbs.

How much can he recover?
Nobody knows, but he can recover function — if he works at it. Recent research studies of brain plasticity continue to uncover promising new information about the three Rs of rewiring: activity reorganizes neural circuits and networks, replaces cells and chemical messengers, and regrows axons, dendrites, and synaptic connections (Dobkin, 2000).

Exercise Benefits for Everyone

Physical Benefits

To help convince your survivor to exercise, remind him that exercise increases physical capacity and ability to perform activities of daily living (ADLs), enhances his immune system, and helps to reverse and control risk factors for heart disease and stroke — high blood pressure, high cholesterol, obesity, high triglycerides, low HDL ("good cholesterol"). Exercise can also prevent or reverse bone loss, help people achieve and maintain healthy body fat levels, prevent or delay serious complications of diabetes, reduce need for insulin, and reduce the risk of colon and breast cancer. Importantly for those with arthritis, it improves endurance, strengthens muscles, and increases joint flexibility and range of motion (CDC, 1999; Elrick, 1996).

> Movement and the functioning of the brain are eminently connected.
> — Rick Rogers

Mental Benefits

These are as important as physical benefits. They include elevated mood, reduced depression and anxiety, increased feelings of well-being, improved ability to handle stress, improved self-image, and intellectual function (CDC, 1999; Elrick, 1996).

Enhances memory. Middle-aged adults who improved their fitness by 15% through cycling also raised their scores on a memory test. Other studies confirmed that cyclists over the age of 55 demonstrate better recall than their sedentary counterparts (Strickland, 1994).

Delays diseases of aging. Your survivor's injury instantly aged him. He's not a candidate for Alzheimer's disease just yet — if he exercises. Exercise can protect him from developing this debilitating brain disease — or at least stay healthy longer. What's the evidence? How about four decades of data on nearly 400 people who engaged in life-long physical activity? (Smith, 1998).

Increases creativity. "Cardio" workouts that elevate the heart rate release chemicals like endorphins, epinephrine, and norepinephrine that promote a positive mood and may also enhance creative thinking. How? Researchers speculate that these opiate-like chemicals release inhibitions which then promote stream-of-consciousness thinking — the ability to think freely and creatively.

Discuss what happens if he doesn't exercise. An inactive lifestyle decreases cardiorespiratory fitness, impairs circulation to the lower extremities, and can lead to osteoporosis — all of which can increase his daily dependence on others, decrease social interaction, and lead to more disability! Inactivity also leads to lower self-concept, depression, and diminished intellectual functioning (Gordon et al., 1998; Elrick, 1996).

If you need still more reasons to convince your survivor to get off the couch, this next study ought to do the trick.

Exercise Benefits for Survivors

To explore exercise benefits, 240 survivors were recruited from various communities in New York. The group of 64 exercisers and 176 non-exercisers were nearly 70% male, ages 18-65, and on the average injured about 10 years earlier. To determine if effects of exercise were different for those with and without disabilities, two non-disabled comparison groups of 66 exercisers and 73 non-exercisers were also included in the study (Gordon et al., 1998).

Exercisers swam, jogged, or bicycled an average of 30 minutes per session, three times a week for six months. While some of the differences between exercisers and non-exercisers were sharper than expected, one finding was a surprise: exercisers were survivors of more severe brain injuries as measured by loss of consciousness. Here are the results:

Overall health. Non-exercisers reported 23 symptoms of health problems significantly more frequently than exercisers. Nearly 35% experienced difficulty in handling personal care versus 8% of exercisers.

Improved physical health. Forty percent of the non-exercisers reported blurred vision compared to 14% of exercisers. Similar numbers were found for waking up and staying awake. Inactive survivors also showed other negative effects — decreased lung capacity and decreased ability to work.

Improved mental skills. Physical activity stimulates the brain and improves oxygen consumption. Continuous movement also requires focus and concentration, which likely results in cognitive improvements. Far fewer exercisers than non-exercisers reported problems in their daily lives — learning, remembering, reading, planning, using time, or seeing others' points of view. *Imagine that*! For example: only 8% of active survivors found it difficult to handle personal care versus over 34% of the non-active survivors, and 20% of exercisers forgot chores versus 52% of non-exercisers.

Improved emotional health. Exercise-induced endorphins really improve mood! Significantly, 34% of the non-exercisers reported feeling depressed versus 13% of the exercisers, 60% felt irritable and nervous versus 40%, and boredom affected nearly 60% compared to 28%. Another study found that of the people diagnosed with major depression, those who exercised and did not take medication improved more than those who only received medication — and those who only exercised did just as well as those who received both medication and exercise (Duke, 2004).

Sharpened job skills. Survivors who exercised reported far fewer problems with being on time, learning, concentrating, organizing, following directions, and remembering. For example, trouble following instructions was experienced by 35% of the exercisers versus 63% of the non-exercisers, and 9% of exercisers experienced difficulty caring for others versus 30% of non-exercisers.

Increased productivity and community involvement. It is no secret that an active lifestyle and community participation are linked — regardless of disability. Exercisers felt less impaired and more mobile and productive, thus leading to better integration into the community. *This means more opportunities for your survivor to feel connected to others and to meet others of the opposite sex!*

Avoidance of the robot syndrome... This set of problems plagues survivors who don't continue to work and is characterized by inactivity, weight gain, boredom, depression, and fear of attempting challenging motor activities (Gordon et al., 1998; Mercer & Boch, 1983).

Typical Problems and Deficits during the Recovery Process

When you read about all the possible problems in this section, you may think that physical activity is contraindicated, if not impossible. Actually not. Your survivor needs exercise even more than non-disabled others because of all these difficulties!

Why? When your survivor is inactive, the negative physiological effects of his disabilities are more pronounced (Gordon et al., 1998). Even if physical activity doesn't improve your survivor's ailments, it can ease some of the depression of being disabled. And the exercise may make him so tired he forgets about the whole disability mess for a while!

Motor Failure

Some time after your survivor's initial injury, as his systems awaken, he tries to move. But as he attempts previous patterns of motion and skills, he soon finds that he no longer possesses the neuromuscular and sensorimotor capabilities to perform them accurately. His central nervous system does not correctly receive, interpret, and transmit information because damaged or inactive pathways distort it. What happens? Failure. Despair. Anger. Try as he might, his body doesn't work like it did.

What are typical sensorimotor and other problems?
Survivors experience several kinds and degrees of problems.

Visual disorders that range from blurred vision to complete blindness are common, as are visual-perceptual and visual-motor coordination problems. If not initially found by medical professionals, spatial relationship difficulties often surface in failed attempts at daily tasks like using keys or inserting coins in slots, inability to find one's way around, and lack of recognition of familiar people.

Vestibular dysfunction is a reduced ability to sense spatial location, due to impaired visual, auditory, and body awareness. Experiencing problems with balance, equilibrium, reaction time, and coordination can lead to dizziness, nausea, fatigue, and headaches.

Vertigo is an imaginary feeling of motion that affects nearly all survivors of moderate injury, and up to ¾ of those with mild head injury. Not to be confused with lightheadedness, vertigo causes sensations of spinning, falling, rocking, and rising.

Other sensory dysfunctions frequently reported include increased or decreased pain and temperature sensation, chronic pain — often from neck and back injuries, sleep disturbances — often an increased need for sleep, and a significant increase or decrease in sexual drive.

Impaired motor function includes problems with movement, fine and gross motor incoordination (ataxia), loss of ability to plan motor movements (apraxia), weakness (paresis) of one or both sides of the body, extremity weakness, abnormal muscle tone and muscle stiffness (spasticity), and seizures.

Diminished physical conditioning and flexibility. The degree of decrease depends on the length of inactivity. Fatigue is common and may be a result of injury-induced factors such as chronic pain, sleep disturbances, hypothyroidism, and depression. Your survivor may also have symptoms of the results of inactivity such as hypertension, diabetes, and heart disease.

Increased susceptibility to both injury and illness. Whether this is due to unrepaired physical damage and/or chemical changes due to head injury is controversial. Because all tasks are more difficult to do, it seems logical that the combination of increased strain, reduced tolerance for stress, and inadequate rest produces injury and/or sickness.

Personal experience. *In addition to numerous stitches, many of the joints, muscles, and bones of my body have been sprained, strained, or broken in the years since my injury, as compared to a few sprains and strains pre-injury. Some may relate this to aging. Nonsense! Most of my injuries occurred between two and fifteen years after my brain injury at age 29. And, based on 12 physical biomarkers for aging, I am fitter than many people half my age! I simply become sick and injured more frequently. In my case, I believe it is due to a weaker immune system, a damaged right side, and decreased coordination, balance, and quickness. When my weaker right side fails, my left side takes the blow and breaks. But reduce my athletic pursuits? — Nah! Sports bring me joy!*

What about his disability and length of inactivity?

Physical disability is not a deterrent. Is your survivor paralyzed? Does he use a wheelchair? These factors are not obstacles to getting a job. Research shows that motor disability does not have a significant impact on rehabilitation or long-term disability. What is vital is cardiovascular fitness and capacity to work. Face it: if he gets tired wheeling across the kitchen to the refrigerator, how likely is it that he could wheel around an office or school or store or repair shop for part of a workday?

Length of time since injury or activity is unimportant. Good news! Studies found that some improvement in functional physical activities can occur long after the injury and initial rehabilitation, even in people whose underlying neuromotor functioning remains unchanged.

Has he been inactive for a while? That's okay, too. These same reassuring studies show that those who have not received intervention for several years may regain lost skills once they start therapy again (Bray et al., 1987; Dordel, 1989). So he just needs to begin — and persevere.

All available research points to the importance of extensive and prolonged retraining — practice! — for any return of function. Neural pathways need to be re-opened and re-energized through repetitive activity. *So, remind him to just do it!*

Exercise Basics

To rewire can be both fun and successful — if he does it right. Help him prepare his physical and mental environments to get fit.

What kinds of activities deliver these benefits?

Any rhythmic movement that continues for at least ten minutes brings benefits. If it's fun, he'll do it!

Outdoor examples include walking, wheeling, Frisbee throwing, cycling, running, skipping, rock climbing, in-line skating, skateboarding, swimming, paddling (kayak or surfboard), body-boarding, and team sports. Work-related activities (such as yard work, gardening, mowing, and carpentry) count too if they're continuous.

Indoor examples include activity classes, circuit training, boxing, martial arts, dancing, exercise machines (treadmill, stepper, bicycle, arm cycle) or sit-down activities (wheelchair basketball, rock climbing wall, chair dancing). Work-related activities count if they're continuous.

When does he start, how vigorous and how much activity?

Now! If not today, when? He needs to start before the "robot syndrome" is added to the rest of his problems. Remind him to wear his scientist hat — to look and listen during his physical therapy sessions.

> You keep on getting what you're getting when you keep on doing what you're doing.
> — Anonymous

Is he having fun? Also consider that 30 minutes of lawn mowing, leaf raking or snow shoveling is equivalent to 30 minutes of wheeling or brisk walking, a 15-minute run, 20 minutes of wheelchair basketball, or 45 minutes of playing volleyball.

Components of a Physical Rewiring Program

Preparation

Locate resources. Contact local facilities to learn about their programs, fees, and if scholarships are offered. Many communities offer free or low-cost activity programs. Explore anything that might be helpful for his continued recovery. Borrow or invest in fitness and strength training books and audio/video tapes. Investigate web sites. Consider investing in a trainer. Find others who want to join him — or a group or class he can join. Check health insurance to learn what it will cover. Be persistent!

Where do we find help?
- Hospital- or community-based rehab centers.
- Colleges — some campuses offer an adapted lab.
- Community/adult education programs.
- Health clubs, gyms, YMCA, YWCA, centers for yoga and martial arts.
- Fitness professionals.
- National and community brain injury foundations.
- Websites for programs such as National Center on Physical Activity and Disability (NCPAD), Disabled Sports USA, Disaboom. See Resources.

Schedule activity, record progress, and reward. Like other important events, remind him to write it on his calendar. Help him keep a record of his progress in a fitness notebook, including daily progress notes. Encourage him to select non-food rewards (or make a treat dependent on achieving a goal), like exercise equipment, outings, etc. — make it his choice! Plan to transport him — or, better yet, join him in activities!

Set goals. Work with your survivor's health-care professionals to help him determine realistic goals. Ask about any limitations, possible medication effects, and warning signs and treatment for overexertion.

Fitness Goals

Before we discuss ways to motivate him — and ourselves — to exercise, let's look at basic fitness goals beyond the enjoyment factor. The primary goal for most people is to "improve health," which includes developing and improving strength, flexibility, and endurance.

As a survivor, he likely needs to add "develop and improve balance and optimism" to his list of goals. It is well known that an improved outlook is a byproduct of a regular exercise program.

A secondary goal could be to "improve appearance." Looking better means losing fat and gaining muscle. Offer to take his photo before he starts his exercise program. Update it every month to remind him of his progress, especially if he becomes discouraged.

Another goal could be to participate in an athletic event — a wonderful opportunity to meet like-minded others. Both indoor and outdoor events occur year-round. "Team-In-Training" programs prepare enthusiasts for a good experience.

The fitness program itself focuses on building strength, flexibility, and endurance. Each program includes three elements: frequency, intensity, and duration. See *Brain Injury Rewiring for Survivors* for more information.

Motivation

Your survivor has decided he wants to be healthier, and to look and feel better. For most of us, participation in activity is based on level of enjoyment, satisfaction, and success. If we like what we do and feel good about it, we do it — if not, we don't. Let's explore how you can help him learn how to overcome any obstacles he might encounter to physically rewiring.

How do I counter his objections?

Beyond enjoyment, motivating himself also involves dealing with some issues. If he has set goals, scheduled activity, and is still reluctant to do it, remind him to use positive self-talk about how good he'll feel. If that fails, try these ideas:

The 10-minute rule. Suggest that he do an activity for 10 minutes. Then, if neither body nor mind wants to go on, he stops what he's doing and asks himself if he needs food, sleep, or a different exercise? At first, he may need to try all the options to find the right answer. Eventually, he will know right away what he needs to do. Basically, he needs to be his own coach — to ask himself what will work to be active.

Change. If he still wants to quit, suggest that he change something else, like his location. Maybe he needs to add music or a companion. Maybe to team together on a work project. Any kind of change can help!

If boredom hits in the middle of an activity, suggest that he change the pace (either faster or slower) or direction. Anything helps!

Rephrase "exercise." Tell him that he's not "exercising"; he's just getting outdoors to see what's happening, neighbors, animals, cars, businesses, etc. Go with him to explore the local park, shops, or malls, or maybe take a road trip somewhere.

Reward exercise time minute-for-minute with something he wants to do — he could exchange activity minutes for video game time. Or make some other activity conditional upon exercise — if he exercises, then he can...

Adopt a dog. He can take it for a walk once or twice a day. And taking care of its other needs can build his self-esteem!

Personal experience. I often used to exercise even if my body didn't want to — then got sick. I eventually learned to take a nap first if I felt tired or didn't want to work out. If I awoke refreshed, I'd follow my plan. If not, I'd go for an easy bike ride or rest more, knowing I'd feel better tomorrow because I didn't push it. Now, I ask myself immediately "Is it food, sleep, or exercise?" and usually get the right answer after I review the past few hours. For example, "I just ate, so it's not that." I also take one or two easy or rest days a week to stay healthy.

What if he's discouraged about learning a new skill?
Remind him that "behavior change precedes attitude change" (Isenhart, 1992). Encourage him to keep going. Frustration often accompanies doing something new. Did you know that moving the memory of a new physical skill to a permanent storage site in the brain may take up to six hours — in non-disabled folks? Researchers found that the first lesson was erased when people tried to learn two new skills within six hours (Liu, 1997) — so suggest that he start with one skill and practice it!

Movement Programs

Many programs have been created over the years to re-educate bodies and minds to promote freer movement. These include Feldenkrais, Hellerwork, the Alexander Technique, and Pilates. In a series of sessions, exercisers practice techniques designed to reduce muscle tension, increase circulation, and change unconsciously ingrained physical and mental patterns of movements in order to improve performance. Other specialized programs (such as Brain Gym) focus on motion to improve brain functioning in the belief that "movement develops intelligence" (Rogers & Brady, 1998).

Despite the ages of participants, most programs begin with functional assessment — can someone roll, crawl, sit, and stand — with and without support. Next, ability to walk is assessed, followed by walking up and down stairs. After mastering these skills, participants attempt advanced techniques like hopping, skipping, jumping, and running.

Feldenkrais

This non-intrusive movement education technique was named after its creator. Trained as an engineer and physicist, Israeli scientist Moshe Feldenkrais developed methods to stimulate proper movement as he attempted to rehabilitate

> Feldenkrais is not just pushing muscles around; it's changing things in the brain itself.
> — Karl Pribram

himself after an old knee injury (Walford, 1997). Imagination plays a part in these specific movement lessons that engage the sensorimotor pathways of the brain. Feldenkrais believed that achieving greater movement increases activation of other mental and physical resources — each stimulating the other.

Functional Integration is a hands-on Feldenkrais therapy in which a practitioner guides body parts with gentle precise movements aimed to integrate the body through simulating the natural exploratory style of learning (Walford, 1997; Wildman, 1986). During a session, people develop new patterns of movement and learn how to reorganize their bodies to operate more efficiently.

Awareness through Movement is a Feldenkrais group therapy in which highly structured motor sequences are verbally directed by a trained instructor. In this technique, parallel to "Functional Integration," group members instruct their bodies to move in ways that will in turn instruct their brains to function at a level that is closer to their potential. The intent of this method is for people to forge new neural pathways through slow, repetitive (20-30 times), tiny movements. Using imagination aids these movements (Walford, 1997; Rosenfeld, 1997).

Who can benefit from Feldenkrais?
Anyone who can move! Whether injured or not, clients learn how to work with their limitations — not necessarily correcting or treating them — to develop more efficient ways of moving. Moshe Feldenkrais believed that most of us use only about five percent of our brain-body potential and that everyone, in a sense, is brain-damaged through non-use or misuse of our brains — whether or not the damage is visible. Some people with motor limitations (such as hemiplegia) who previously had little hope, showed dramatic improvement (Wildman, 1986).

Hellerwork

Joseph Heller developed this mind-body technique that combines deep tissue muscle therapy, movement education, and massage. To help realign the body and release chronic pain or stress, clients follow a specific sequence of movements while engaged in a structured dialogue with their practitioner. The aim is to gain insight into the memory or issue that is the underlying cause of the tension (Natural Healers, 2004).

The Alexander Technique

Developed in the late 19th century by F.M. Alexander, this is considered the "grandfather" of movement re-education techniques. This mind-body method to understand coordination is practiced by observing habitual patterns of movement and then self-correcting by eliminating those that are unnecessary. Alexander discovered that the head literally acts as a steering wheel for all body motion by moving ever so slightly (Engel, 2004).

Pilates

This mat exercise technique combines calisthenics and yoga to improve flexibility, strength, and balance. Recently popular as a new way to develop core strength, "mat work" was actually developed in the 1920s by Joseph Pilates when he was interned in England during World War I.

To help rehabilitate those he nursed, Pilates devised equipment using bed springs. Today's equipment is remarkably similar to the early design with back and neck supports, spring tension, and straps to hold hands and feet. As a complement to mat work, sessions with a trained teacher to develop abdomen, buttocks, and back using precise slow movements designed to enable a new awareness of muscle function and control (Pilates Method Alliance, 2004; Pilates, Inc. 2004).

Personal experience. A program featured in my local newspaper was recommended by professional athletes so I paid attention. The premise of this approach is that the body is naturally designed to work smoothly as a unit. The program's focus was to re-align our bodies through relaxing, strengthening, and stretching so that functioning will return — or at least improve. I signed up for four sessions and still refer to The Egoscue Method of Health through Motion *(Egoscue & Gittines, 1992) as I learn to trust the wisdom of the body.*

What equipment is helpful?
While high-tech apparatus is beneficial and fun for your survivor, lack of access to a rehab center does not mean his improvement needs to stop. Daily practice with basic equipment promises greater gains than once-a-week training on high-tech devices and it doesn't need to be expensive to work. The key? Practice-practice-practice!

Mobility training: Lying or kneeling on a scooter board is useful and fun. This apparatus can be a skateboard-like device or a small box with large casters and a cutout for one leg. Weights can always be added for more resistance (Torp, 1956).

Balance work: Build or purchase the spring-a-ling, a trampoline-like device constructed from two 3' square boards with heavy-gauge springs at the corners (Wahlstrom, 1983). A balance board can be constructed from a 1' x 2' x 1½" piece of hardwood that sits on two 3" wide x 3" thick x 10" long wooden half-circles. This can be made wider, lower to the ground, and/or covered with carpeting. For a balance disk purchase a 3' disk of wood and cut a space for a softball.

To work on both balance and flexibility and to have fun, your survivor can lie on a large balance ball, rolling forward or backward or in other directions to play!

Assistive devices support injured limbs and provide stability for walking, balancing, and lifting. Walkers, canes, crutches, braces, and prostheses improve mobility. When your survivor begins balance activities, he may feel more secure with a supportive device such as a horizontal bar attached to walls, posts, or even a chair or table. As his skills develop, he can gradually diminish his use of a support — for peace of mind, it helps to have something to grab, if necessary. Custom-made shoe inserts (orthotics) equalize legs of different lengths and help support feet and legs. If gripping is a problem, limbs can be strapped to equipment with elastic or Velcro wraps.

Why is practice so important?
Studies show that functional motor skills may have to be relearned in much the same way as originally learned (Rinehart, 1983). According to experts, precise practice must occur — thousands, even millions of times — in order to successfully perfect the motor pattern (Kottke, 1980).

Although brain plasticity allows the formation of new synapses during learning, practice may be required for months — or even years — before new synapses develop and function (Rinehart, 1983). To exasperated objections to his practice paradigm from survivors like me, Dr. Kottke replied, if it took three million steps to learn to walk, why expect that it would take any fewer to re-learn to walk?

Relaxation Activities

Several activities provide techniques for relaxation. Your survivor may find any or all of them helpful.

Yoga

Yoga is the spiritual tradition from which the healing Ayurveda emerged. Although we Westerners view yoga as a gentle strengthener for the body and calming technique for the mind and spirit, as traditionally practiced it is a complex system of exercise, diet, and philosophy. See *Brain Injury Rewiring for Survivors* for more information.

Qigong

You've likely seen Kung Fu and Tai Chi movements practiced, but maybe did not know that the grounding concept behind these systems is Qigong, which literally means "the meditation practice of Qi energy." The name is derived from the

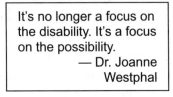

It's no longer a focus on the disability. It's a focus on the possibility.
— Dr. Joanne Westphal

Chinese characters *qi* meaning universal bioenergy and *gong*, which represents the effort placed into *qi*.

Developed 4,000 years ago in the cold and damp region along China's Huang River, locals who did what was called "the big dance" stimulated the acupuncture meridians and did not succumb to the aches, pains, and illnesses normal to this climate (Evans, 1997).

Accessible Gardening

Encourage your survivor to use the natural world and gardening activities to enrich his body, mind, and spirit. Confronting obstacles and finding creative solutions is a liberating process.

Ultimately, both people and plants bloom!
— Holden Arboretum

Perhaps a green thumb connects to a blue ribbon — and maybe not. Either way, hands get dirty and hearts get warm. Anyone who's planted a seed or seedling learns about growth and life. Your survivor nurtures it with food, light, and water, and watches it grow and blossom, satisfied and joyful with his efforts that resulted in such a product! Yes, it is indeed sweet to see the fruits of our labors — and they are edible.

And anyone who's seen his plant wither and die — or not even germinate — also learns about death and loss. We can sit and sulk or rise and explore what didn't work and why — and try again. The miracles of growth also encourage psychological healing and social development as interactions about nature and gardening naturally occur — a perfect rehabilitation setting!

Accessible Gardening guidelines:

- **Paths.** Make paths at least 36" wide. Raise beds 4" to 27" off the ground, accessible from both sides and up to 4' wide.
- **Watering.** Using a pulley system is easier than watering cans.
- **Easier moving.** Use discarded coolers set on dollies
- **Horizontal planters.** Construct these from PVC pipe using old pots for end caps and wire them to a fence or mount on wooden legs.
- **Vertical garden.** Use wire, a discarded plumbing pipe for support, and two wooden pallets to construct a "sandwich." Drive the pipe into the ground and wire the wooden pallets on the outside. Line with black plastic. Fill with soil-less mixture — lighter than soil. Make slits in the plastic for seedlings (Hair, 1999).
- **Adaptive Tools.** Lightweight hand tools affixed to the end of a long handle extend reach without the usual bending and kneeling. Padding for handles can be easily created from foam rubber or pipe insulation. Ergonomically designed products such as "Handform Trowel" allow your survivor to dig into the soil without needing a tight grip on a tool. A "cut and hold flower gatherer" facilitates cutting and retrieving flowers at any height. To locate these tools, see your local garden centers, adaptive catalogs, or the Holden Arboretum website.

My Recovery Journey Experience

At the time of my injury (1976), physical and occupational therapy for moderate head injuries was not offered. I was told, "You're not bad enough" when I requested help, despite my problems with right-sided weakness, balance, visual-perceptual coordination, speech,

> Flowers always make people better, happier, and more helpful; they are sunshine, food, and medicine to the soul.
> — Luther Burbank

headaches, and total body pain! Although medical authorities — and insurance — offered massage for my black-and-blue back twice a week, two of these sessions provided more than enough pain, so I declined any more.

What did I do? Well, after numerous outbursts relocated me to the psychiatric ward, I decided that the medical community was not going to help me. Duh! So, after my last hospital release, I began my own rehabilitation program at the local gym.

For more physical rewiring, I also enrolled in activity classes at the local community college. These included tennis and golf, which my body wasn't ready for yet, and karate, for which it was. I also played softball with a low-level recreational team. As a collegiate athlete, it was not especially gratifying to play at this level, but it was where my skills fit. I could still be a star, it was fun, and I liked my teammates.

What else did I do? Swimming! In desperate need of independence again, about eight weeks after my injury I moved back to my apartment building, which was blessed with a swimming pool. Lucky for me, my father — a former coach — came over every day after work to swim with me. He not only knew how to motivate me — "Do one more [lap] than you think you can do, Honey" — but he wanted to be with me, which survivors know is not that common.

Bicycling! Although doctors told me I wouldn't be able to ride my bicycle or play tennis, naturally I didn't believe them. However, after many erratic attempts and a few falls, I believed them — for a while. To relearn how to ride, I decided I needed a more user-friendly bike, so I purchased a mountain bike with wider tires and an upright position.

Do I still fall? Yep — but I'm falling less and it sure beats driving! During the over thirty years since my injury, I have crashed a number of times, injuring nearly all of my body part, but not my brain — thanks to my brain-bucket helmet! Crashes are the price I'm willing to pay to feel the sun on my face and wind on my back. I also feel much safer and happier riding a bike than driving a car, so I ride — and compete in triathlon and duathlons, in off-road and track venues — they're all fun!

Running! I found running to be one of the most difficult sports to relearn. After persevering with minimal success for eighteen years, I finally analyzed the problem — coordination! Finding an understanding coach who advocated special drills helped me to look more like a runner, but I'm still not fast — I just look and feel better and actually like it now!

In-line skating! I'd never seen a skater with fat legs, so I decided to try this sport to improve coordination while saving my joints. It's fun, gives a good workout in a short amount of time, is not difficult to learn, and can be fast or slow. It does require a bit of daring — no problem, right? Ski poles with rubber tips give my arms a good workout and aid balance.

Board-surfing! Learning to surf was a goal of mine for several years after I moved to San Diego. After trying several boards that didn't fit, numerous crashes, little fun, and no professional instruction, in 1994 I found a coach, a board that fit, no major crashes — and I began to enjoy myself! I stood up on the very first day, and gradually felt more confident as I went through three lessons and eight weeks of practicing. My balance deficit still hampers me but I congratulate myself after small successes, and the ocean is a soothing and forgiving medium. My brain and body don't always do what's needed, so some days I surf smaller waves, but that's okay — "small steps lead to success." I know I have to "pay my dues" to learn.

Body-board surfing with fins is fun, easy, and a good workout!

Kayak surfing! What to do when most surfing adventures find me on my butt? Buy a sit-on-top kayak! I still fall — but it's a shorter distance and easier to climb back in and catch another wave.

Strength training! Even when injured, enough of me always worked well enough to sit and lift weights — and if I worked hard enough, I could even get a "runner's high."

Yoga and stretching! A gentle voice to guide me, peace and calm — that's been my yoga experience. Whether in a large class or small, I always enjoy the gentle work and feel better during the rest of my week. Yoga is a deceiving workout — it feels harder than it looks.

My Hope for All of Us

I hope and pray that your survivor too will utter the "I will" and "I can" words. Maybe he won't say them at all — he'll just do it! Or he may refuse to do anything at first. Encourage him, be a role model, ask him to join you. Soon you'll hear, "Okay, I'll try." Then you've got him!

> Movement and the functioning of the brain are eminently connected.
> — Rick Rogers

Gradually he'll come to find enjoyment in activity and the camaraderie of it. Joy is contagious! Later, perhaps, he'll initiate being active — or maybe not. He's still trying to accept his new physical state. Keep searching for fun ways to engage him physically and emotionally. I promise it'll work!

Summary

- Believe that exercise benefits survivors in a big way!
- Know that length of time since injury or previous activity is unimportant.
- Understand that if it took three million steps to learn to walk, why would take any fewer to relearn to walk?
- Help set him up to succeed before he starts.
- Encourage him to do physical activities he likes every day.
- Remind him to schedule his activities.
- Investigate programs that improve his movement.
- Explore accessible gardening and relaxation activities.
- Seek places that offer help with physical activity.

> You can't cross a chasm in two steps.
> — Rashi Fein

11
Social Rewiring:
Healing Spirits with People Connections

Treat people as if they were what they ought to be and you help them to become what they are capable of becoming.

— J. Van Goethe

With the injury, your survivor's social skills took a hit along with his head. In the electrical nightmare that was created, some embers smolder, others ignite, and still more erupt. Sparks are common.

You've witnessed — and experienced — the combustion that arises from the faulty circuits. You probably don't recognize this new behavior, feel helpless, and want to do something.

Introduction

Your survivor, too, probably asks himself, "Who is this crazy person in my body?" He's also confused by others' responses to him.

This chapter will help! Knowing about social deficits and related behaviors, you can explain to him that his current social problems result from what he does rather than what he is.

As you observe the sparks, you can work with the rewiring team to analyze the sources of the "shorts." Then together you can reinforce frayed filaments, replace outdated switches, reroute circuitry, rebuild connections, insulate all wires — and maybe even reduce the current to avoid overload! With everyone linked, positive energy can replace negative. He can relearn social skills!

This chapter covers:

- Social skills deficits.
- Psychiatric and cognitive connections.
- Behavioral, emotional, and social connections.
- Loved ones' response to behaviors.
- Relationship changes.
- Loved ones' stress, coping strategies, and resources.
- Post-injury dating and sex.
- Helping your survivor relearn communication skills.
- Helping your survivor relearn behavioral and social skills.
- Programs and strategies to improve behavior and social skills.

First, he says, "Okay, world — here I come!" Then — gripped by fear — he decides that maybe he's not quite ready, despite all his hard work. He subsequently reconsiders this, saying that he's tired of waiting and if no one appreciates him the way he is, then that's their problem. What happens? Like anyone else with social problems, he's ostracized. And this isolation extends beyond the neighborhood gathering — it affects all of his life. In fact, many studies show that survivors' social and interpersonal skill deficits interfere more with community living and productive employment than any other consequence of traumatic brain injury (e.g., Burton et al., 2003; Prigatano, 1995).

Social Skills Deficits

What are social skills deficits? What behaviors are likely to occur?
"Social skills include relevant knowledge of social rules, roles, and routines; effective perception of social cues; a repertoire of situation-specific behaviors; and settled dispositions to act in ways that achieve desired social outcomes in chosen social contexts." These skills can be divided into "competence skills" — knowledge of rules, roles, and routines, and "performance skills" — the ability to act on the knowledge in real social situations (Ylvisaker 2001).

In other words, just because someone knows what to do doesn't mean he can act as if he knows, or maybe he just doesn't want to be socially correct. If that's not it, then other factors — such as not accurately reading cues, being impulsive, or showing no interest — can lead to social awkwardness. If environmental factors such as noise and activity are added, is it surprising that survivors appear socially inept?

Social skill deficits and their common related behaviors are seen in these areas:

- **Personal:** self-centered behavior, decreased motivation, decreased tolerance for frustration, decreased self-control, impulsive behavior, poor judgment, inability to self-monitor and correct behavior, decreased ability to learn from experience.
- **Interpersonal:** impatience, dependency, socially inappropriate behavior, increased irritability, insensitivity to others, temper, outbursts, and sexual disinterest or preoccupation.
- **Environmental:** increased sensitivity to noise (especially loud and sudden), blinking and flashing lights (from laser pointers to strobe lights), multiple conversations, other movement, and surrounding activity — basically anything that invades a survivor's space without permission is considered an alien force.

These coping and functioning difficulties can create problems that are easily misdiagnosed as psychiatric. And by their very nature, the typical lesions caused by brain injuries produce a combination of cognitive and personality problems that are not seen in non-injured people or in those with identified psychiatric disorders (Prigatano, 1987).

Complicating the challenge for one and all is that survivors show extreme variation in deficits due to the difference in injuries as well as their pre-injury personalities and coping styles (Tate et al., 1991).

Let's look at three candidates for the mentally ill label, any of which can cause social miscues: cognitive lapses, emotional and/or behavioral reactions to cognitive lapses, and other emotions that compound the errors!

Cognitive Deficits

Cognitive skills are the link between mental skills and social action.

Returning World War II veterans who had sustained brain injuries in combat provided the first clues to this link. Dating back to 1942, scientists discovered connections between personality changes and damage to the brain and its cognitive functions when they reviewed test results. The same soldiers who acted in socially inappropriate ways, often impulsively, also performed poorly on abstract reasoning problems (Prigatano, 1987).

Memory disturbance and lack of inhibition are closely related to personality change and are often cited by experts as related to social dysfunction. Competency in interactions is further marred by impairments in flexibility and expectations that others act out of their same worldview. Survivors also find it difficult to transfer skills and to generalize in new situations. What is the cumulative effect of multiple failures? Distress, loss of self-esteem and self-confidence — in addition to loss of job opportunities and friendships (Tate et al., 1991).

Survivors' communication difficulties — particularly in interactive conversation, verbal memory, and learning — are key to predicting ability to return to work and full community participation (Stein et al., 1995).

But there is good news! Those dysfunctional behaviors that are associated with cognitive impairment can improve along with better cognitive function even many years after injury (Namerov, 1987; (Thomsen, 1992).

Which cognitive deficits interfere with social skills?

While survivors demonstrate a diverse and selective pattern of neuropsychological impairments, probably the most noticeable deficit is in *executive function*. Socially adept people are proficient in this multi-tasking skill in which their inner executives plan, organize, direct, and control tasks and interactions — while observing and responding to non-verbal cues from others.

This *executive-function* deficit is perhaps the most disabling consequence of brain injury because survivors can't see it. Survivors may appear competent in their demeanor, yet because they're unable to monitor, evaluate, and alter their social behaviors, they don't self-correct (Vogenthaler, 1987). Likely many survivors get in trouble because they don't read body language at all or perceive it incorrectly. In other words, they don't "see" cues.

Those with intact social skills employ their executive function in conversation all the time — automatically! Socially competent people look at a speaker, accurately read cues, and remember previously successful behaviors to appropriately respond in a timely fashion. Despite unpredictability and variability, they know what to do and say.

Part of your survivor's stress in responding in a conversation is "time urgency" — a need for him to say what he means in a reasonable length of time. Other barriers to communication include cognitive inflexibility, slowness of response, and language deficits.

Basically, the difference in processing communication between survivors and uninjured others is comparable to using a manual versus automatic transmission in a car. Survivors need to precisely analyze a situation to decide how to act. Although their conversational skills may never be automatic again, they can flow more smoothly. Just realize that your survivor now "drives" a manual transmission — and his goal is to improve social interaction — it's do-able with lots of practice.

Behavioral, Emotional, and Social Connections

"What's wrong with the way I'm acting?"

Does this sound like your survivor? Not wanting to admit there's a problem with his behavior is typical. This post-injury refusal — it's not denial in the psychological sense — is thought to be due to a more complex disturbance in self-perception and self-awareness (Prigatano, 1995). Your survivor doesn't "see" what's wrong and is frustrated that he can't do what he did and is unable to control his emotions.

The cause of this changeableness or emotional lability is the damage to the frontotemporal lobes and to the limbic center that normally controls emotions. With the acceleration/deceleration forces in motor vehicle accidents and repercussions from contact sports and bomb blasts, it is suspected that some functions are depressed and some are sensitized (Mamelak, 2000) — no wonder it's so confusing for everyone!

Your survivor's behavior reflects his feelings — the more distressed he is, the more he exhibits disturbed behavior. As one of his loved ones, you've no doubt experienced his inability to control anger and other strong emotions, as well as his difficulty identifying and expressing his feelings.

Anxiety and depression — internally experienced as misery and externally exhibited as hostility — are common emotional symptoms for many survivors. Others see the outward manifestation of their inner pain (Hoofien et al., 2001).

Can anything be done?

Yes, improvement — even many years after injury — is possible. Social skills can be relearned even 20 years and possibly more after injury (Thomsen 1984; 1992).

Skilled therapists work with survivors to restore previous capacities and skills and to compensate for permanently impaired abilities. "It is easy to become entangled in pragmatic variables and forget an obvious but often forgotten dimension: Our clients are persons, and thus they have the inherent capacity for modifying behavior" (Malkmus, 1989).

This approach works for me! Rewiring social skills is just another kind of rehabilitation, isn't it? A skill is a skill. Just as your survivor regains competence in other areas, so can he relearn how to be more socially adept — with your help.

Loved Ones' Response to Behaviors

In the early post-injury stage, loved ones typically respond to their survivor with enabling behavior — joy that the survivor is alive causes understandable relief that then leads loved ones to ignore, accept, tolerate, or simply manage behaviors that would have been unacceptable pre-injury.

And physical rehabilitation demands so much energy — from everyone — that little attention is paid to poor behavior — until it doesn't go away! Loved ones may not want to put too much pressure on the survivor for fear of upsetting him. Consequently, many survivors are allowed to get away with murder — almost! — Just because everyone is glad that they're not dead!

This glee fades with time. When inappropriate behavior doesn't stop or improve, others may become angry with the survivor or avoid him altogether. Former friends gradually visit and call less often, family members want and need to get on with their own lives — and the survivor still doesn't know what he's doing to drive people away!

What to Do — Soon after Injury

Question your survivor about social experiences, both pleasant and unpleasant. This may prompt him to initiate behavior training on his own. He may seek answers to others' words or actions.

> He has the right to criticize who has the heart to help.
> — Abraham Lincoln

Later, likely it will become necessary to confront him with what happened and why — particularly if an inappropriate behavior has been ignored and unquestioned for a period of time. If he denies it:

- Set up scenarios — perhaps in a joint therapy session with a counselor — to practice the different interactions.
- Develop mutual cues to use in public:
- Set timing policies — when to offer suggestions to him.
- Give control to him. "Is this a good time to tell you…" — If he says, "No," honor it and ask again at a later time, saving you both the aggravation — and the outburst.

What to Do — Later after Injury

Use SAFER

Stop. Before venturing out, inquire if he feels ready — rested, fed, mentally and physically prepared, etc.

Assess. Upon arrival, observe the noise and activity level of the place. Ask him if it's acceptable. If it is, be attentive to signs of distress — cumulative effects can make it intolerable, whether he notices it or not.

Survivors may try to deal with this before they're ready. Continue to monitor if he's okay. As soon as he verbally or physically expresses a need to leave, immediately GO! Survivors often miscalculate how much distress they can handle and are over their threshold quickly.

Fix/Evaluate/Retry. If the environment is not acceptable, ask him if he wants to move to a quieter section or request a volume reduction. If he wants to leave entirely, then explore what to do next. Later, discuss what happened, what worked and didn't work, and what steps to take next time.

In addition to SAFER:

Set yourself and your survivor up for success. Before attempting a conversation, especially one that may be hard for him to hear, ensure that his physical (food, sleep, exercise) and emotional needs are met.

Display patience. Perhaps the most important listening skill for loved ones is patience. He can better communicate — and is less likely to argue — if he feels valued and is not pressured about time.

Suggest options. When he's ready, suggest optional ways of doing and saying something. Incorporate the SAFER plan here.

Relationship Changes

Marriage

Like a pebble in still water, brain injury has ripple effects beyond the initial contact site. The closer to the impact, the more the damage is felt. If a marriage is involved, in addition to harm to two separate people, the relationship itself suffers loss.

Disturbance replaces homeostasis. The sense of balance between two people is forever altered. From physical and financial interdependence to agreement about children, careers, and lifestyles, a marital union is about accord. Couples make a link because the various puzzle pieces fit together at enough critical junctures for the relationship to work. If one or more pieces change shape slightly, the other pieces mold to fit — no big deal.

But a brain injury *is* a big deal. It upsets everything! This major event changes not just the puzzle pieces, but also the board itself. Nothing remains unscathed. Discord invariably occurs. When uncertainty replaces stability, worries replace dreams and frowns supplant smiles.

"I didn't agree to this!" shouts the non-injured partner — in vain. No one wants the disruption of a brain injury. Whether you accept the changes or not doesn't alter the fact that they occurred. The new puzzle pieces can form a workable pattern again — but with a major reorganization of roles and expectations, and an acceptance of the new puzzle in its dynamic state.

To re-shape pieces that are established and comfortable is a challenging and complex process. Just as your survivor journeys through the grieving cycle, so does the marriage, with similar breakdowns, detours, and stops along the way.

As in any relationship, communication is the key. Not only is it important that both partners acknowledge the differences created by the injury — how it has affected your survivor and also the marriage — but also the strengths of the relationship — the glue that holds the couple together. Integrating these two themes can positively affect the marriage and help it to remain intact (Sher, 1997).

Often the task seems too daunting. Despite efforts and regardless of the love involved, some pieces just don't fit anywhere, while others link on only one side. Those pieces left on the table overnight seem to change shape and color entirely! Many factors cause failure of the post-injury marriage puzzle. Injury not only destroyed the old puzzle pieces and board by changing shapes, sizes, and even colors, it also created a new board. Can the redesigned pieces connect to form a new, workable pattern? That is the challenge! The marriage as it was is now a memory.

How many post-injury marriages succeed?
Good news! A recent study found that the great majority of couples remain married! Only 17% of 120 survivors of all brain injury categories divorced and 8% separated between two and one-half and eight years after injury. This finding refutes previous dire reports that most of these marriages fail.

Two factors important to stability — the length of the pre-injury relationship and severity of injury — were confirmed in earlier studies. Found to be unrelated to marital breakdown were gender, ethnicity, educational level, time since injury (previously reported as important), and post-injury employment status (Kreutzer et al., 2007).

Other factors improve post-injury marital stability: if survivors are older persons whose injuries were non-violent, whether children are involved and their ages, and degree of support — family therapy and a social network.

Previous research found that the percentage who divorced following brain injury varied from 5% to 49%. In a study in Israel of 76 married survivors between 10-20 years after severe head injuries, the rate of divorce was 5% (Hoofien et al., 2001). A UK study reported a rate of 49% for 131 survivors within a 5-8 year period of injury (Wood and Yurdakul, 1997). Why the difference? Hoofien et al. suggest the discrepancy "may reflect cultural differences in coping and attitudes towards disability or differences in sampling."

How do post-injury marriages succeed?
In addition to the length of the relationship before injury, researchers suggest that marital stability may be due to an adjustment of expectations by the non-injured partners, 87% of whom are female (Hoofien et al., 2001). These spouses compared the new relationship to that of a parent with total decision-making responsibility, which is incompatible with the role of sexual partner (Gosling and Oddy, 1999).

And while the Israeli marriage rate was over 64%, family members reported feeling a high sense of burden and stress that increases over time, a finding that was confirmed by other studies. Not surprisingly, having good social support means less psychological distress. Without this assistance distress increased with time after the injury (Ergh, Rapport, Coleman, and Hanks, 2002).

Even though satisfaction with family functioning was rated positively by both survivors and family members in these studies, Gosling and Oddy (1999) reported that all non-injured female spouses rated marital satisfaction as significantly less than their male partners — primarily due to major role changes — and that the only positive aspect of these relationships was a continuing sense of commitment and companionship.

Another way to view changed intimacy is presented by Donald Kautz in *Hope for Love: Practical Advice for Intimacy and Sex after Stroke* (2007), suggesting that partners of survivors "...separate caring for from caring about" to help maintain romantic feelings despite caregiving responsibilities. Planning intimacy for times when both partners are well rested and experimenting with different positions, activities, and aids during sex play can also increase satisfaction.

Recent research concluded that both partners need to develop three problem-solving strategies for marital adjustment following brain injury: an effective attitude towards problems, infrequent use of avoidance tactics, and a positive perception of one's spouse's communication skills (Blais & Boisvert, 2007). The good news from this research is that both survivors and loved ones can learn these strategies!

Family

Families rank the change in social behavior as *the* most stressful consequence of brain injury — more stressful than differences in cognitive or physical abilities.

Emotional Responses

Either guilt or responsibility for the injury may be felt by siblings, depending upon the survivor's position and status in the family. Siblings may also feel neglected by parents who focus most of their energies on the survivor and resentful that they now must assume new chores, responsibilities, and different roles within the family. Survivors often feel jealous of successful brothers and sisters.

If the survivor still lives with his parents and siblings, they all may be angry that he disrupted the flow and integrity of the household by returning as a different person. Experiencing a wide range of emotional reactions and feelings about their new situation is normal. Thus, non-judgmental acceptance and voicing permission to express and discuss these feelings is important (Grinspun, 1987).

Because more interactions take place within the family than any-where else, family therapy is vital for everyone's mental health. To return to equilibrium, some experts suggest that a goal for families be adjustment rather than acceptance, as they work through the stages of grief outlined by Elizabeth Kübler-Ross (See Chapter 6.) Going through each stage requires everyone to adapt. Family members may not like or accept changes, but working together — not in isolation — to successfully incorporate those changes builds a stronger family unit. Part of the adjustment involves non-injured siblings not subordinating their needs to satisfy the perceived needs of the survivor. If that occurs, everyone loses (Sher 1997).

Relationship Patterns

Like other life events, post-injury sibling relationships face three possible outcomes: better, worse, or no change. Your survivor's previous personality and the nature of his relationships accurately predict both of these after injury, which intensifies tendencies.

If relations were difficult before, then it's probable that these same dynamics will persist afterward. It is also likely that most of the repair work, if it's chosen, falls on the non-injured family member, whether out of guilt or responsibility.

Friendships

We can say that more than internal wires shorted with your survivor's injuries. Connections to some old friends, as well as family members, fizzled and frayed. If we view the family as a mirror of society, we can expect similar responses from friends as from family members. After the initial post-injury rush to his side, avoidance is common. Sad but true, that is what happens, as many survivors will attest. Explaining some possible reasons for their responses might help your survivor understand, especially if you help him grow. He can make friends again!

Losing — and changing — relationships conflict with our search for dependability in all things. We like sameness, especially with loved ones. How many of us can go with the flow and accept that relationships — like life — are dynamic? What if only one person is dramatically changed? Because this "new" person may look like the one they used to know, it is difficult for people to express something no one wants to admit: perhaps they liked the "old" person better. At the very least, they *knew* the "old" one. No one knows this new person, including the survivor himself. Some loved ones may be unable to continue their association because of the change.

As your survivor's necessary post-trauma egocentricity gradually diminishes, others may be able to relax and be involved in a more mutually satisfying relationship. And, as he grows toward interdependence, he can consider the needs of loved ones as well as his own. As the years pass and he becomes an interesting new person, some of his pre-injury friends may return — or they may not. If he continues to grow, he will attract others into his life who didn't know him before and like him as he is now. *Isn't this a relief for everyone to know!*

Strategies
After your survivor's chosen memorial service (discussed in *Brain Injury Rewiring for Survivors*), seek new connections with your survivor, not just helper-helpee links: activities that you mutually enjoy. Perhaps take a class together that interests both of you or explore something new. See the Survivor's social chapter for activity ideas and ways for him to make new friends.

Post-injury friendships
Not just pre-injury friends find it difficult to sustain a relationship with a survivor. In addition to his uneven social skills, similar companionship challenges emerge as people mature and grow in different directions, whether old friends or new.

Strangely enough, your survivor's progress can cause problems if he continues to develop — and they don't. Some may be threatened by his growth and choose not to continue the friendship. For example, if they were first attracted to him because he needed them and now he doesn't, the relationship no longer offers rewards, so the friends move on.

Words of wisdom from my post-injury best friend, Marlys Henke:
"Here are some of my thoughts on being a friend of a survivor:
- You must like the survivor enough to just deal with the disabilities. If you can see the Divinity within the survivor — the good, the

peacemaker, the oneness with the universe — then all else is just details.

- Take a guilt-free break to do your stuff — go see violent adventure films, or go dancing with flashing disco balls, or whatever you enjoy that the survivor can no longer do. It is not necessary to adopt all his life-style limitations. If you do, you will eventually resent being the martyr.

> It is only with the heart that one can see rightly; what is essential is invisible to the eye.
> — Antoine De Saint-Exupery

- Remember that the survivor has no choice about not being able to screen out loud noises, flashing lights, or whatever sets off his brain, so be protective.
- Support whatever the survivor feels successful doing. The activity or its usefulness is not the point. Feeling successful at something is the critical issue.
- Let the survivor do what he can for you — give gifts, do chores, whatever — so that the relationship has some balance and is not all you-give-and-they-take. Also, if you can help the survivor do socially appropriate acts like bringing a small gift to a dinner party, this will help recovery.
- Slow down and wait for the survivor to catch up — physically and/or mentally. This will be good for both of you!
- Set up a schedule for being together — talking, eating, or doing an activity — so you don't get overwhelmed by his neediness. If needed, this also helps the survivor relearn how to set and respect limits.
- Praise is absolutely necessary and needs to be repeated often. Help the survivor develop positive self-talk to help pull himself out of depression and disappointment.

I give thanks for our friendship every day!
Love and Namaste, Marlysis"
(We added "sis" to her name because we "adopted" each other!)

If former relationships included drugs and alcohol, what can loved ones do?

Help him find purpose and friends again. Just as with non-injured folks, those with meaningful relationships and activities don't need to fill a void with chemicals. Investigate local resources, including groups for those with disabilities, for activities and recreational services. Community colleges, adult education, and YMCA/YWCA often offer programs. Your survivor needs to be actively involved with rehabilitation of all kinds. See Resources for more ideas.

Eliminate environmental cues to use substances. Keeping him substance-free may include removing alcohol from your home or storing it in an inaccessible location as well as limiting access to funds to buy it.

Refuse to accept that he needs to use alcohol or drugs to belong or because "everything else was taken away." Remember that deficits from the injury already place your survivor in a group that is likely to be suspected of intoxication by local police — slurred speech, unsteady gait, poor memory, volatile moods. Adding a substance simply increases the likelihood of run-ins with local authorities. Remind him, too, that his cognitive deficits can result in being fooled into buying herbs like oregano instead of marijuana, so he also loses his money! (Falconer, 1997).

Provide your survivor with a "Survivor Identification Card" — available from The Perspectives Network (see Resources). This will help others understand common symptoms of brain injury and to ensure your loved one isn't arrested for intoxication!

Stress and How to Cope with It

Research has found that the amount of stress experienced by family members largely depends upon time since injury, severity of injury, and the survivor's neurobehavioral disturbances. More burden is understandably felt by those whose survivor showed the most disturbed behavior (e.g., Wood and Yurdakul, 1997; Ergh et al., 2002).

Overall, a moderate level of distress was felt by family members. This "dis-ease" and sense of burden, which increases over time, is often expressed in anxiety, hostility, depression, and physical illness (Hoofien et al., 2001). Anxiety and depression are primarily felt by spouses or parents (Ponsford et al., 2003); anger and fatigue are the main symptoms when males are involved as caregivers (Perlesz et al., 2000). Loneliness despite support of pre-injury friendships was also noted (Wedcliffe and Ross, 2001). Not surprisingly, due to the burden, families are at increased risk not only for divorce, but also for substance abuse and economic instability (Albert et al., 2002).

In addition to survivor personality changes, another crucial factor in family members' stress levels is how these changes are perceived. Not knowing what to expect and how long social deficits take to improve exacerbates these levels (Grinspun, 1987). Seeking professional guidance and involving yourself in the rehabilitation process can help to replace feelings of helplessness and hopelessness with empowerment (Jacobs, 1989). Supportive counseling also helps families to better manage these feelings. (Also see Resources for books devoted to the family).

***Personal experience.** In keeping with the Midwestern culture and the "we don't talk about it" era of the 1970s, as well as the few services available, my family did not participate in a support program. Even with my inability to read subtleties, their facial expressions revealed their feelings — and my religious heritage told me it was my fault. Undoubtedly, their distress would have been greatly eased, and my recovery hastened and less painful, with some kind of family support. Because nothing was said, I felt cut off from family affairs, further estranged from one sibling, and more distanced from the other. Unfortunately, with the pattern set, we still don't talk about these feelings more than thirty years later.*

Strategies for Families and Other Loved Ones

Let's review concepts about stress before we discuss how to reduce it:
- Realize that stress is personal and cumulative.
- The impact felt from the same stressor may be different at different times, depending upon overall stress level.
- Accept that stresses — and your responses — by themselves are not either good or bad.
- Avoid judging yourself and your body's responses.

"Okay," you say. "I know that we need to rewire our family. How do we do that?"

Here are some steps to lessen the burden and manage the stresses, converted into challenges to overcome (Falconer, 1997). And remember SAFER!

- **Identify stress**. List all daily tasks; include those things done for everyone in the family — not just your survivor. Rate these items on a scale from one to ten, where "1" signifies no stress and "10" means high stress — where anything would be more fun!

- **Reduce or eliminate stressors**. Decide which regular tasks rated over "5" actually need to be done. Then analyze: can they be done another way, less frequently, or at a different time of day? Can someone else do this task — like the survivor, a friend, another family member? Focus on only those things that are meaningful and do them efficiently. With the time saved from reducing and eliminating, you can replace stressful situations with pleasant ones!

- **Maximize capabilities** of others, including your survivor. Be specific when asking others to help: inform them exactly what is needed, when, how often, and what you can offer them in return. Evaluate with your survivor what tasks he can do and ask him to suggest how he can independently do those tasks routinely done by others for him. For example: change the time of day something is done, schedule more time for it, provide all necessary materials including written directions and/or pictures to allow him to complete tasks independently. Experiment! Provide opportunities for both stress reduction and growth of everyone!

What coping resources are effective for families and loved ones?

Social support — whether it is professional or non-professional (friends, family, religion, support groups) —not only enhances family functioning, but also decreases caregiver distress (Wedcliffe & Ross, 2001; Albert et al., 2002). Adequate social support even helps those whose survivors showed severe cognitive and behavioral dysfunction and whose injuries were not recent — factors that otherwise caused increased caregiver distress (Ergh et al., 2002).

In addition to face-to-face contacts, support provided by telephone is also effective, as demonstrated by a "social work liaison program." Results showed that families caring for survivors with all types of brain injuries reduced caregiver burden in many areas (such as anxiety, inadequate sleep, low energy, isolation) and increased satisfaction with the care-giving role and mastery of that role. In this program, loved ones maintained telephone contact with the same social worker initially assigned in the hospital. Counseling — both individual and family — was the service most requested, regardless of whether loved ones initiated the call or social workers phoned (Albert et al., 2002). Other options include respite care for you and transitional living and independent living programs for your survivor.

What programs offer help to both survivors and loved ones?
A community-based program that provided peer support for both survivors and family members enhanced overall quality of life and ability to cope with post-injury depression, while improving general outlook (Hibbard et al., 2002).

One family support program addressed everyone's needs. In this multi-component intervention, services for survivors included cognitive remediation, emotional adjustment, social competency, and behavioral retraining. Families received a structured program of education to satisfy their need to know about brain injury; communication skills and problem-solving training to reduce family strain; and case monitoring, support groups, crisis intervention, and information referral to reduce the demands on loved ones.

All participants reported high levels of satisfaction with this program six months and two years post-injury. Important benefits reported by loved ones included declines in distress over survivor symptoms, lower levels of depressive symptoms, greater levels of self-esteem, and less use of physician services (Smith & Godfrey, 1995).

If family programs aren't available, survivor-only programs are also successful. Imagine 89% of former severely behaviorally challenged survivors living successfully in their home communities three to four years after implementation of behavioral supports! And costs decreased in the first year of community integration (Feeney et al., 2001).

Survivor Dating and Sex

Dating after injury

While it's different from socializing before his injury — and more complex — the reasons are the same. If your survivor chooses to date, then he does so with a disability. He can view dating skills as part of his rewiring or he can sit home with the remote. What's more appealing to him? (Remind him that social isolation leads to more depression.)

Will others want to date him? It depends — is he attractive to others? Remind him to look nice, demonstrate good manners, show an interest in others, and display a sense of humor. His desirability is probably related more to personality and character, leisure pursuits, and career plans than to any particular disabling feature. And, importantly, does he like himself — and others?

Consider that it is your survivor's disturbed behavior that creates social problems — not intellectual or physical qualities. So, encourage him to seek help with behavioral areas and then to venture out and socialize. The more he practices, the better he'll get. For sure, the more he stays alone, the worse he gets! He can date and find compatible soul mates!

Sex after injury

As surprising as it seems in this age of disclosure, little has been reported by experts about sexuality after TBI (Zasler & Horn, 1990; Eliott & Biever, 1996). If sexual alterations and dysfunction are discussed, studies generally focus on the incidence of dysfunction, rather than how to fix it. Sexuality management, treatment, and strategies for survivors and their partners have been largely ignored — even with sex listed on the what's-changed list. So, this rather disinhibited author presents the what, why, and how about sex after injury in *Brain Injury Rewiring for Survivors*.

Relearning Communication Skills

Environment is vital to this area of his recovery, too. A relaxed setting, patience, and conversational prompts from interested listeners show your survivor that others value what he says, will wait, and will help him say it.

While it's a challenge to overcome the barriers to communication — cognitive inflexibility, slowed response, and language deficits that are common to brain injury — regular intentional practice helps.

> The first big task of interdependence is thinking and understanding each other — that means talking together.
> — R. Bellah

Conversation Improvement Programs

Using a social cognitive approach can improve competence. These programs focus on the different parts of conversation: purposes and features, interpretation of both speakers' intents and listeners' reactions, and how to achieve specific conversational goals. Varied speech acts, such as requests, are also practiced.

This approach is especially helpful for two groups: those who were injured before these skills and information were acquired (children and adolescents) and those who lost their abilities and skills for interpreting social behavior.

These programs could be used in many settings, from one-on-one at home or in therapy to a group setting such as a support group. If you choose to coach at home, see the "Cognitive Rewiring" chapter for reminders about how to learn and teach a skill.

The following section incorporates descriptions from both *Head Injury Rehabilitation: Developing Social Skills* (Burke, 1997) and *The Conversation Improvement Program* (Ylvisaker, 1997).

Decoding skills: what did they say?
The abilities to receive, understand, and interpret or translate information are often called decoding skills. Any injury that damages the ability to break the code may result in behavior that is erratic, impulsive, or constricted. An inability to decipher such information interferes with socially competent performance. If your survivor doesn't speak the language, he can't talk with those who do! The solution is to learn,

practice, evaluate, and then practice again. Use video or audio tapes. Choose any or all of these:

Help your survivor gain awareness of conversational features:
- **Identify** the various parts of conversation on any topic: opening, maintaining, taking turns, extending, shifting, and closing.
- **Discuss the rules** of conversation and possible reasons for this code of conduct. For example, why do people take turns when they talk?
- **Role-play** different types of conversations. Discuss the appropriateness of different patterns such as balanced and uneven turn taking.
- **Practice** ways to extend and shift the conversational topic, like open-ended questions that ask for opinions — "What do you like/think?" extend discussion — "Oh, that reminds me," and shift or change the topic.

Help improve his ability to interpret speaker intent:
- **Discuss** the speaker's intent and possible interpretations. Identify and evaluate reasons to support your view. Point out distorted inferences, especially patterns.
- **Role-play** conversations under various kinds of speaker intentions: Practice ways to encourage, sympathize, threaten, insult, inquire, and entertain. Identify various signals of meaning, including body language, proximity to listener, and facial expression.

Help him gain awareness of conversational topics and rules:
- **Identify topics** and trace the flow. Discuss relevance of each contribution, and effectiveness of any attempts to control.
- **Role-play** conversations. Open, maintain, control, and change. Vary the settings. Use open-ended ("What did you like...") and "why" questions to extend the topic and seek information.
- **Practice** techniques to open, interrupt, and shift topic: "Oh, that reminds me..." Practice ways to close conversations and use markers to indicate interest: "Yes, go on."

Help develop his ability to utilize various speech acts:
- **Practice** techniques for different conversational intents — how to give and request information, direct, assert, demand, refuse, warn, promise, compliment, criticize, tease, joke, comfort, encourage.

Help develop his awareness of listening behaviors.
- **Role-play** situations with various listeners — those of different ages, abilities, and familiarity to the speaker. Discuss appropriate techniques for each.
- **Practice** how to read and infer the listener's interest in a topic. Discuss how to see the listener's comprehension and emotional reaction both to the words and to the speaker.
- **Executing skills**. "Did I say that right?" and "Come again?"

Help develop his effective speech and listening skills:
- **Review, role-play, and rehearse** rules and social/cultural mores:
  - Maintain comfortable physical distance, eye contact, and interested posture.
  - Use polite words.
  - Refrain from certain topics and use of certain words in public.
  - Speak clearly and at an understandable pace.
  - Don't talk with anything in your mouth.
  - Practice strategies to repair conversational breakdowns as both listener and speaker: "Could you repeat that, please?" "I don't think I understand." "I'm not sure I said that right. Let me start again…"
- **Role-play and critique** conversations that utilize all the various speech acts and rules:
  - Give information, request information, direct, demand, assert, refuse, warn, promise, compliment, criticize, tease, joke, comfort.
  - Observe how the response was received. Repeat.
- **Practice** saying clearly and concisely what you mean.

Summary of the five steps in the reply process:
- Receive stimuli.
- Consider ways to respond.
- Evaluate the likely consequences of each action.
- Select the best choice from your repertoire.
- Deliver your remarks.

Relearning Behavioral and Social Skills

To become socially competent again, survivors need to intentionally relearn social skills. As with any new skill, practice improves ability to perform. Therapy or volunteering in a real-world setting provides good places for your survivor to work to regain skills.

Community Agencies

Opportunities to practice social skills abound! Historical, cultural, and health-related agencies often seek greeters. If that sounds too scary to him, suggest other kinds of work in healthcare settings — help to play with children and aid in teaching various adaptive activities such as swimming are often needed, as is help to deliver mail and beverages. If face-to-face meetings are too stressful, other opportunities such as answering telephones, stuffing envelopes, filing, or fixing things can provide limited practice. Survivors usually feel comfortable in health care settings because they've spent a lot of time there!

If your survivor prefers to interact with animals, contact local humane societies and animal shelters. They often welcome willing hands and hearts for a variety of tasks from cleaning cages and kennels to rescuing. If the outdoors beckons, then trail and ground maintenance could be a choice, trees and flowers often need planting, etc. Even with minimal contact with other humans, he's reentering the community and gaining some social skills practice as well as feeling valued. Everyone wins!

Requirements. Time commitment varies with the agency. After a brief training period, as little as three or four hours per month may be enough. Some agencies require a specific weekly pledge of time, while others' needs correspond to the season or event. For example, food banks need people at the Holidays, people and animal shelters need extra help during cold weather, etc.

Programs and Strategies to Improve Behavior and Social Skills

We know that improved cognitive functioning results in greater emotional control and supports my plea: *"Fix my brain and I won't be crazy!"* Survivors with improved cognitive function can also function better in the community.

> Behavior change precedes attitude change.
> — Mary Alice Isenhart

Cognitive-neuropsychological skills.

When survivors are satisfied with their cognitive functioning, their renewed sense of self-efficacy translates into improved community integration. This conclusion was drawn after survivors completed a four-month, highly structured rehabilitation program that integrated cognitive and psychosocial interventions. It is an especially hopeful finding because it related to survivors who had been previously unable to resume community functioning (Cicerone et al., 2004).

Cognitive-behavioral skills.

Survivors with extreme behavior problems who participate in an intensive, integrated, and individualized program including real-world social situations can learn socially competent behavioral habits and apply them in their community. Components of such a program include support by various professionals and communication partners, elimination or reduction of negatively provoking events, alternatives to problem behavior, developing a positive sense of self through daily practice, regular use of effective medication, choice and control in daily lives and social interactions (especially to avoid negative and/or difficult social experiences), meaningful/interesting/doable tasks, and positive roles and scripts (such as personal heroes).

Identity mapping is integral to this program. In this activity, a survivor selects two metaphors: one that represents his current thinking and feelings, and one that positively reflects work and strategies to be successful in school, work, and social life.

After extensive research and more than 30 combined years of experience working with survivors with cognitive, behavioral, and communication disorders, this program was developed to answer the need for something that works! (Ylvisaker & Feeney, 2001).

Does time since injury affect rehabilitation success?

No! This is good news! Even many years after injury, participants in a multidiscipli-nary community-based outreach rehabilitation program made significant gains that continued past the active

> Limited expectations yield limited results
> — Susan L. Willig

treatment! Survivors aged 16-65 who had sustained severe TBIs between three months and 20 years previously participated on an average of twice a week in community settings for an average of 27 weeks. Follow-up measurements of 48 survivors, taken at an average of 25 months after treatment, included self-organization and psychological well-being as well as level and activity of participation in the community. Results showed that 40% made clinically significant improvements (Powell et al., 2002).

What general behavioral strategies are effective?

When problem-focused approaches are used, good things happen! Post-injury, many survivors use ways of coping that don't work. Researchers who asked 74 survivors and their family members about ways of coping found that less use of emotion-focused, avoidant, and wishful-thinking tactics predicted better survivor psychosocial functioning (Malia et al., 1995). And, when family members used problem solving and behavioral coping strategies after TBI, the survivor had significantly lower levels of depression (Leach et al., 1994). *I bet the family members did, too!*

Social strategy do's and don'ts (Ylvisaker & Feeney, 2001):

Employing action-oriented strategies helps all survivors set themselves up for success, whether they display extreme problem behaviors or not. With your survivor and others in his daily life:

Do:

- Identify specific obstacles to social success and strategies to overcome them (time of day, setting, people present, etc.).
- Identify specific social goals and strategies to achieve them.
- Use daily routines, people, and places to practice social skills because they are situation-specific.
- Provide support for positive interactions in specific situations, then withdraw it as soon as possible when it's no longer needed.
- Create success-producing activities, especially before any stressful events, e.g., ask him to do something he does well.
- Develop specific interactive scripts for all communication partners for stressful interactions.
- Create numerous opportunities for coached practice.
- Eliminate situational provocation for habitual negative behaviors.
- Be flexible about plans and strategies to avoid confrontation. Change time, day, etc.
- Reward positive social behavior with natural social consequences.
- Follow negative social behavior with natural social consequences, such as removing him from the setting.
- Create opportunities for your survivor to play important roles as a "non-disabled" helper and responsible person.
- Seek opportunities for natural interaction with potential friends.
- Create opportunities for safe satisfaction of sexual desires.
- Consult with specialists about appropriate medications.
- Be patient! Life-long patterns of thinking, feeling, and acting change slowly.

Don't:

- Excuse bad behavior in an attempt to understand it.
- Expect that training and/or behavior from clinical/restrictive settings will generalize to everyday social situations and contexts.
- Expect consequences to mold or guide future positive behavior.
- Use consequences to organize plans for behavioral and social situations — your survivor may not remember what he did.
- Impose your values on your survivor or others in his sphere.
- Demand strict compliance with planned interventions.

- Assume you can control everything in another's life.
- Forget to remind your survivor to respect others' rights and needs. Say: "You are not alone in this world; others are important, too."

Tips from my post-injury friend Diane Rennell:
You know your survivor friend is overloaded — internally or externally or both — when he:
- Says or yells, "Wait! Wait!" in a conversation.
- Becomes stuck on something previously said in a conversation.

The best strategies are to:
- Honor her discomfort and "wait." Allow your friend to go back to what she's stuck/intent on.
- Jog her memory with cues if she doesn't remember saying and/or doing something.

Survivors often find it difficult to measure others' intimacy needs and thus may be too touchy-feely, without mutuality. If this behavior is noticed in the company of others, gently discuss it later, providing cues to remind your friend of what transpired (Rennel, 2004).

Your Survivor and Activities with Family/Friends

It's no secret that all living things require nourishment to grow. Those who are injured or sick benefit even more than others from a stimulating environment. Not only is increased activity and social interaction a natural and logical part of any recovery, it is essential because:
- Neurotransmitters respond to external influences such as interactions with others. People really do need people — a good connection can usually reverse a bad mood instantaneously!
- The focus is on an activity or project, rather than just on skill improvement (*which gets real old!*), and includes others with mutual interests.

What kinds of activities?
Anything your survivor is interested in is a good idea, regardless of its usefulness. Work-related and productive activities naturally follow his

increase in self-confidence and involvement with life and others. See *Brain Injury Rewiring for Survivors* for ideas.

Summary

Although your survivor may never return to his former sociable self, he can rewire his skills. Remind him of these concepts:

- His social difficulties result from what he does, not what he is.
- He can learn new behaviors because all brains are adaptable.
- Not all social glitches result from his mistakes.
- The dysfunctional behaviors caused by cognitive impairments can improve with better mental function even years after injury.
- He needs to do whatever feels successful.
- Rewiring social skills is just another aspect of rehabilitation.
- Social interaction is essential to recovery.
- Incorporate the SAFER plan into social activities.
- Affirming and welcoming people and places do exist.
- Keep knocking on doors to find these people and places.

Remember:

- Develop mutual cues to use in public.
- If you expect certain behaviors, your survivor needs to know what to do.
- Give control to him.
- Eliminate environmental cues to use substances.

> When you get to the end of your rope, tie a knot and hang on. And swing!
> — Leo Buscaglia

- Know that counseling helps families better manage their feelings.
- Reduce or eliminate stressors related to household tasks.
- Maximize capabilities of family members, including your survivor.
- Believe that post-injury marriage can succeed — with lots of work.
- Social support decreases stress and is vital for family functioning.
- Social skills/conversation improvement programs are effective.
- Programs and strategies can improve behavior and social skills.
- Follow social strategy do's and don'ts.

12
Vocational Rewiring: Healing with Productive Activity

How many doors do I have to knock on?
> — Author

As many as it takes.
> — Psychologist DJ

You've probably heard your survivor say something like, "Work? Why would I want to do that? Who needs work to be happy?"

He does!

Introduction

Research shows a very strong connection between employment/ productive activity and quality of life. To be fulfilled, people need to be productive. And if we do something meaningful, we don't need to retreat into unhealthy habits. Finding purpose enhances recovery — fleeing into substance use derails it. This chapter looks at the following areas:

- Value of work/productive activity.
- Benefits of volunteer work.
- Return to work/productivity — what are my survivor's chances?
- Internal and external success factors for return to productivity.
- Effective work and vocational service programs.

- Government programs that help support your survivor.
- Obtaining retraining/education.
- Electronic memory devices for job success.
- Getting fired/not hired.
- Self-employment.
- Handling rejection.

Value of Work and Productivity

Work is one of life's essentials. It gives people a way to use their time productively, structures each day, and provides a place to be sociable.

> The grand essentials to happiness in this life are something to do, something to love, and something to hope for.
> — Joseph Addison

Importantly for your survivor, productive activity not only provides meaning and purpose, it also offers a setting to re-establish a social life. Community re-integration and return to productive activity are interrelated — research found that the improvements in social adjustment were largely confined to those who worked (Oddy et al., 1985).

If your survivor is not productive, he faces the same problems as anyone else who's unemployed — unstructured time, no opportunities to show competence, and no source of identity or network of friends.

Benefits of Volunteer Work

It is no secret that personality and ability to get along with others are often the best predictors for successful community reentry (Prigatano, 1987). At volunteer work sites, survivors can practice and improve elusive social and work skills in hospitable environments with accepting people such as senior citizens. These mutually helpful relationships offer emotional connections that benefit not only your survivor, but also provide respite for you and his other loved ones and caregivers. Good news, indeed!

At the same time, your survivor reenters the community in a productive way, helping to restore precious self-esteem. Volunteer work provides opportunities to be the helper rather than the one being helped.

A win-win situation that we can call workplace interdependence occurs when everyone's needs are met (Condeluci, 1996).

Personal experience. When I served as chairperson for the San Diego County Disability Awareness Week Network (DAWN) in 1991, we worked toward two goals: raising awareness of schoolchildren and influential adults in the community and motivating them to make needed environmental and attitudinal changes.

Brave, able bodies played the roles of those with various disabilities for a period of time ranging from five minutes to several hours. And a wheelchair obstacle course provided a good photo opportunity for courageous politicians. As a result of their experiences, good things happened! When a city councilmember attempted to take public transportation to an event, the wheels of his wheelchair lodged between trolley rails as he tried to cross the street. Maintenance crews soon corrected the problem!

Our lobbying local celebrities and politicians to participate paid off in extensive media coverage, including nightly television highlights, several newspaper articles, and mention in the Congressional Record. Participating in our event was an in-thing to do!

Where can your survivor volunteer?
Virtually any organization — including virtual (Internet) — seeks volunteers. Whatever your survivor wants to do is wanted somewhere by someone. He can search by worksite such as animal shelters, recreation centers, and telephone hot lines, or by work preference such as manual or technical, or by location such as indoors or outdoors, or just by special events. See *Brain Injury Rewiring for Survivors* for details.

Return to Work/Productive Activity

Good news! Most survivors return to productive activity (RTPA) after their injuries. Although my review of 28 studies from 1990 to 2004 found return to productive activity ranged from 25% to 96% for all survivors, many factors affected these results. Additionally, some research considered only paid work. See the review in the *Brain Injury Rewiring for Survivors* Vocational chapter.

You may wonder: why such a wide range? What else does the research show? Let's examine:

- Factors that can predict the chances of return to work (RTW).
- The likelihood and rate of return to work.
- Occupations where survivors usually work.

Factors that Predict the Chances of Return to Work

Age

Researchers generally conclude that age is an important factor in influencing outcome. More severely injured survivors return to work if they are injured in their late teens or early adulthood than if injured earlier (Askainen et al., 1996) or later in life (Kraus et al., 2000). Possible reasons for this include less neuronal reserve and increased likelihood of complications and associated injuries in those older than 50 years (Kayser-Marcus et al. 2002). For survivors of mild and moderate injuries the role that age plays is variable, depending upon other factors. Studies differ regarding the impact of age.

Gender

Women fared better than men in return to work or school despite experiencing less recovery in all outcome categories, according to a review of all available data (Kraus et al., 2000; Farace and Alves, 2000).

What are possible reasons for gender differences in outcome?

Researchers suggest that any of these may apply: the effect of the mechanism of the accident (women were usually injured in motor vehicle crashes, as pedestrians, or in falls), treatment variables such as effects of medications, or pre-injury sex differences (Farace & Alves, 2000).

Outcome may also be affected by basic gender differences in brain physiology, including baseline differences in brain metabolism — women have higher cerebral blood flow and increased neuronal processes. Sensitivity to estrogen cycling is also a factor in animal studies: estrogen is protective in male rats but exacerbated brain injury in female rats (Kraus et al., 2000).

What are possible reasons for gender differences in return to work?
Why do women return to work despite poorer outcomes than men? The difference may be related to cultural role expectations. For example, it is socially acceptable for women to take on a dependent role but not so for men. Brain injury creates a period of necessary dependency — thus mandating that men try to forget or overcome their cultural conditioning to accept a needy role.

Perhaps women used vocational rehabilitation services to a greater degree. Are women more able to adapt to circumstances and change careers? Are they more willing to work and go to school part-time? Are women injured at an older age and thus more highly educated and engaged in a career pre-injury? Are they more willing to work in typically lower-wage jobs, such as in service industries?

Another possible factor is that women return to work *despite* physical complaints. In one study, 73% of 67 survivors of mild-to-moderate brain injury returned to work despite significant symptoms, including headache, fatigue, and forgetfulness/poor concentration. Those who failed to return to work reported cognitive and behavioral complaints (Vander Naalt et al., 1999). However, because this research did not differentiate between genders and men sustain more injuries (3:1), can we expect that men also overcame these same complaints to return to work? It is also possible that some types of work reported for women (such as homemaking) — and not for men — accounted for this finding.

Substance Abuse

Research shows that survivors with no history of pre-injury substance abuse were more than eight times as likely to be employed at nearly two years post-injury (Sherer et al., 1999).

Education

Survivors with education beyond high school who are injured in late teens or early adulthood typically achieve better vocational outcomes than those with less education, regardless of injury severity.

Occupation

The level of pre-injury employment plays a role in RTW. A survivor who returns to a higher-level occupation can use a greater range of skills and enjoy greater decision-making latitude and a more flexible employer (Kayser et al., 2002; Ruffalo et al., 1999).

Severity of Injury

Research shows that, however measured, RTW is strongly related to severity of injury: the worse the injury, the less chance of return to paid work. This doesn't mean there is *no* chance your survivor can eventually earn wages nor does it mean your survivor will not be productive in some capacity! In fact, survivors of severe injury who participated in rehabilitation programs achieved an employment rate of 50-65%, whether measured short or long term (Hoofien et al., 2001).

Types and Degrees of Impairments

Kinds and severity of deficits also impact return to work (West, 2001). Although many survivors are employed in some capacity, they may need to work fewer hours or with fewer responsibilities or at a lower salary than pre-injury. The effect of impairment on a survivor's likelihood of returning to a previous job depends in part upon the nature of the pre-injury employment. For example, returning to any occupation that relied on vision, such as driver, electrician, librarian, or surgeon is unlikely with visual deficits.

Studies Measuring Return to Productivity

Research shows that most survivors return to productivity after their injuries, so keep the faith. A community-based survey found a rate of 78% for 107 survivors of 71% severe, 18% moderate, and 11% mild injuries. For 29% of these, their injuries occurred 10 or more years previously; the average time since injury was 7.1 years and the range was one to 30 years. Of the actively engaged 78% of survivors, 18.6% worked for pay (5.6% professionally) or attended school full-time, 59% worked (paid or volunteer) or attended school part-time; some did both! (Dolen, 1991).

Another study found that 9% to 23% work full-time (depending on region), another 10% to 19% work part-time, 15% sought work, 40% volunteered at least once per month, and 15% attended school or training. As expected, the percentage of full-time workers decreased post-injury: the percentage of all survivors who work full-time dropped from 75% pre-injury to 9% in the East and 23% in the Southwest. Previous full-time workers decreased to 63% for more mildly injured survivors (High et al., 1995).

Rate of Return to Paid Work

Research showed that the percentage of survivors who work for pay, either full or part-time, slowly rose over a period of at least ten years after injury (High et al., 1995). When viewed by injury severity, a study of 366 survivors found that 38% of those with severe injuries, 66% with moderate, and 80% of those who sustained a mild injury returned to paid work within two years of injury (Dikmen et al., 1994).

More typical results (for less than two years): 72% of 105 survivors (64% mild-moderate) returned to paid work at 1-year post-injury, doing the same or comparable work (Wagner et al., 2002) and 42% of 50 mild TBI survivors returned to paid employment (12% at the same level and 30% modified) at six to nine months post-injury (Ruffalo et al., 1999).

Rate of return to work for those with severe injuries.

Overall, return-to-work percentages varied from 30% to 61% for survivors with moderate to severe injuries, depending upon study location and job description. An Australian study of 208 survivors two to five years post-injury found that 38% had "returned to a high level of productivity" (Doig et al., 2001).

Forty-three German survivors of severe injury defied their prognoses when 30% of them were able to continue successfully with their previous jobs! In a seven-year follow-up study, 37% reported a stable return to work at pre-injury levels and 16% at a lower level, which means that a total of 53% returned to gainful employment (Possi et al., 2001)!

Long-term vocational status was reported in a Canadian study and it is impressive! Fully 55% of 131 male survivors of severe injuries returned to the same level of full-time employment as pre-injury

(Stambrook et al., 1990)! Over six years post-injury, 59% of 44 American survivors of moderately severe injuries were employed in some capacity. Of these, roughly half reported working fewer hours or with fewer responsibilities or at a lower salary, compared to pre-injury (Burton et al., 2003).

In an Israeli study 10-20 years after injury, 60% of the 76 survivors of severe injury were employed at the time of follow-up. Although the majority (73%) worked in low-level unskilled jobs, 61% of the survivors were employed in competitive jobs, while 39% worked in either sheltered or volunteer settings, an average of 14 years post-injury (Hoofien et al., 2001).

Surprisingly, one study of 304 moderate-to-severe survivors reported a figure of 29% for full-time workers, which is phenomenal! Significantly, the study included survivors up to 24 years post-injury (Colantonio et al., 2004).

In a study that reported employment stability, of 186 American TBI survivors who were employed pre-injury, fully 61% were employed between one to four years post-injury. Of these, 34% were stably employed and 27% were unstably employed at three follow-up intervals. "Stable" represented employed at all three follow-ups and unstable meant employed at one or two of the follow-ups (Kreutzer et al., 2003).

In which occupations do survivors usually work?

Little data is available about employment areas. Consistent with their need for structure, survivors of severe injury often work in the fields of technology and administration. Especially at their lower levels, these fields involve structured, routine tasks that don't require initiative or creativity. Combining this with little need for social interaction makes both fields particularly good fits for survivors of severe injury. A small minority, including those with mild injuries, find success in work that is more creative and in socially demanding fields (Hoofien et al., 2001).

While some highly educated survivors return to professional positions, those able to work full time declined after injury from 32.7% to 5.6%; those working part-time increased from 2.8% to 4.7%. Post-injury workers in the trades include 8.4% both full and part-time, declining from 36.4% and 9.3% pre-injury (Dolen, 1991).

Warehouse, clerical, and service-related occupations provide employment for the majority of persons in a study of supported employment (Wehman et al., 1993).

What about job stability and long-term productivity results?
Another obstacle to achieving true vocational rehabilitation is the employment instability of survivors. To advance at work usually requires steady employment for prolonged periods of time, more than survivors' average employment of 3.5 years (Hoofien et al., 2001). Rehabilitation programs can significantly improve their stability.

Good news about long-term productivity! Significant improvement in cognitive, vocational, motor, behavioral, social, and interpersonal functioning occurs between two and over 10 years post-injury, according to close relatives of survivors of severe injury (Sbordone et al., 1995).

How can loved ones improve survivors' work success?
Realize that your life and that of your survivor were forever changed by the injury. Not expecting him to be the way he was — and not complaining about your life now — enables him to be the best he can be at any time. If others appreciate him as he is, he can, too.

Know that he will change over time, his progress will be uneven, and that setbacks are natural. Know, too, that regardless of the severity of the injury, he has a capacity to learn. Practice and training in physical and mental exercises result in improvement.

Adopting a healthy lifestyle and habits is good for you and him. Learn what works and stop doing those things that don't work! Ask him and others for ideas how best to help. Give him constructive feedback — one idea at a time — with his permission.

Avoid giving your survivor advice that may contradict that of others. The best way to know what he's heard is, if possible, to ask him rather than the sources of the conflicting advice. Discuss the different points of view, considering each as an alternative. Then develop a plan that your survivor can endorse, using the SAFER method. Remind each other that many solutions are possible for a problem! But do realize that your survivor is likely confused and frustrated at trying to do what one person says and then learning that someone equally valuable to him disagrees!

Support his choice — whatever it is — and respect each other so a united front is presented (Kreutzer & Kolakowsky-Hayner, 2001).

Family members can also help their survivor just by being productive in their own lives! A Taiwanese study of 85 participants found that the number of productive members in the family was one of three influencing factors in post-injury employment status, with average rate of return to work at least six months post-discharge of 81% (86% mild, 79% moderate, 58% severe) (Chen & Howng, 1994).

Success Factors for Return to Productivity

External Success Factors

For a survivor to succeed in a work environment takes more than motivation. Important factors include returning to the same job and/or employer, flexible work scheduling, environmental modifications,

> It is not fair to ask of others what you are not willing to do yourself.
> — Eleanor Roosevelt

health insurance, and a socially inclusive atmosphere (West, 2001).

Several environmental factors also affect survivors' workplace success. When audio and visual distractions are reduced or eliminated their competence increases — they need some degree of control over external stimuli. Other controllable job features, such as multiple demands on attention and need for rapid processing, can also jeopardize performance (Montgomery, 1995). Mild TBI survivors found success when they returned to positions with greater decision-making latitude and social interaction on the job (Ruffalo et al., 1999).

Remember, too, that regardless of the setting, survivors demonstrate inconsistencies in performance, between tasks, days, and even hours of a day. *Never a dull moment!*

Internal Success Factors

How important is getting along? — It's vital! Personality and psychosocial variables are often the strongest predictors of successful community reentry, according to numerous studies (e.g. Prigatano,

1987). Survivors probably have new behaviors that get in the way. They need:
- Capacity for acceptance.
- Self-awareness.
- Ability to regulate emotion.
- Functional independence.

Capacity for acceptance is the single most important factor in predicting return to work. For 59 survivors of moderate to severe injuries who participated in a 20-week intensive neuropsychological remediation program, acceptance meant that they complied with program routines, objectives, and staff recommendations; actively participated in the community; and publicly acknowledged problems (National Institute for Disability-Rehabilitation Research, 1994).

Acceptance doesn't require employment. For 78 survivors who were one to two years post-injury, those with active unemployed lives reported a higher Subjective Rehabilitation Status (SRS) than others who were unemployed with passive lifestyles. Although both groups showed a lower SRS than those who worked, both employment and SRS were related to acceptance of disability, although which comes first is not known (Melamed et al., 1992).

What is acceptance?
Irrespective of time post-injury and more than a stage achieved, acceptance is a continual process of ebb and flow. Immediately after injury, survivors' typical denial and lack of self-awareness result in a kind of acceptance, but it is short-lived and easily short-circuited. Attempts to deal with it can result in depression, substance abuse, and other unhealthy behaviors. The realization that this is what it is comes gradually.

What you can do.
You can help to convince your survivor that each person has an intrinsic, God-given goodness and that, despite injury-caused impairments, this essence and wholeness cannot be destroyed by any amount of damage to

the body or mind. Help him to connect with others who value him for who he is and not for what he does or how much money he makes.

Effective Work and Vocational Service Programs

Supported Employment

For people who are disabled and beginning to return to work, this is the most effective placement technique (Wehman et al., 2003). When survivors participate in such therapeutic work programs, 50-70% of them reenter the competitive work force, compared to an unemployment rate of up to 90% with no intervention (West, 1995; Haffey & Lewis, 1989).

What is supported employment?

Supported employment is a way for people with disabilities to work for pay in competitive settings in the community. Various kinds of ongoing support services are provided to both employers and employees, such as job coaches, individual supervision, assistive technology, and specialized job training.

Job coaches help in several ways. In addition to providing specialized on-site training to workers, they are available to employers for help in dealing with challenging behaviors and for periodic consultations with co-workers and employers. They also give orientation training to co-workers, if needed (US Dept of Labor, 2005).

Supported employment success

Productivity rates of 67%, 75%, and 87% are reported! The 67% productive activity rate applied to 80 severe-injury survivors who were at least five years post-injury (averaging six years). Comparing months worked to the number of months available to work during a five-year time period, they improved from 13% with no services to 67% with supported employment, working in warehouse, clerical, and service-related occupations (Wehman et al., 1993).

One group of 41 survivors with severe injuries worked 75% of total available months in competitive employment after receiving services from an on-site specialist, compared to 15% before, with job retention of 71%! (National Institute for Disability Rehabilitation Research, 1994).

The 87% productivity figure was reported for 101 survivors who averaged 5.5 years post-injury and participated in a Medical/Vocational Case Coordination System (MVCCS). They received medical and vocational rehabilitation, work trials, and supported employment services, including job coaching. Injury severity rates included 21% mild, 7% moderate, 56% severe, and 16% undetermined. At the 1-year follow-up, 53% were involved in independent work, 19% in transitional placements, 9% in supported, and 6% in sheltered work, while 13% were unemployed. Vocational independence at the initial placement predicted employment status at follow-up. Those with greater disability required more extended time and more extensive rehabilitation services before placement (Malec et al., 2000; Malec, 2005).

Social Security Ticket to Work Program

Those who receive federal disability benefits — either SSDI or SSI — may participate in this vocational service program. Ticket to Work aims to increase opportunities and choices for people to obtain employment, vocational rehabilitation, training, job referrals, and other support services so they can achieve their vocational goals (Social Security, 2005, 2007).

State Vocational Rehabilitation Agency

As part of the Ticket to Work Program, your state agency can provide various services for education or training, including financial assistance.

> Satisfaction lies in the effort, not in the attainment. Full effort is full victory.
> — Mohandas Gandhi

Day Treatment Program

All survivors who participated in the Comprehensive Day Treatment Program at the Mayo Medical Center (Rochester, MN) achieved impressive results. Injury severity rates included 7% mild, 7% moderate, 82% severe, and 4% undetermined (too long post-injury to recall). At one-year follow-up, 67% of the 96 program graduates were productive. Averaging 4.6 years post-injury, 39% were engaged in independent work, 10% in transitional placements, and 18% in supported or volunteer work.

Importantly, all survivors improved their participation in society, whether injured six months or "many years" earlier (Malec, 2001; 2005).

Equally as impressive is data from another Minnesota rehabilitation program for 44 TBI survivors with severe neurobehavioral disorders. Graduates of this rehabilitation program not only improved and maintained their gains at a three-year post-discharge follow-up, but 50% of them were employed at least part-time (Murrey & Starzinski, 2004).

Neuropsychologically Oriented Rehabilitation

The goal of this multi-faceted program is to use a social context to improve cognitive and emotional functioning and quality of life. When survivors are involved in this type of rehab that includes mental retraining exercises, they change their attitudes toward work and a higher proportion return to gainful employment — 50% treated vs. 36% not treated. Just as important, according to relatives, participants experience less difficulty with "emotional adjustment" to the injury (Prigatano, 1995).

Governmental Programs

Social Security — SSDI and SSI

Government disability benefits provide a lifeline for survivors. Apply as soon as possible after injury. Either phone the Social Security Administration (SSA) office (800-772-1213) or use the website www.ssa.gov/disability. If you call, the number will be busy. **Keep calling!** You can determine his eligibility for all Social Security programs by completing the BEST screening tool on the website. Two federal programs pay disability benefits: Social Security Disability Income (SSDI) and Supplemental Security Income (SSI).

To qualify for SSDI: Either the survivor is at least 22 years old and has paid into the FICA system when he worked for qualified wages or he was disabled before age 22 and his parent(s) paid into the system or his parent receives either disability or retirement benefits or is deceased. Average earnings determine monthly payment amount. **Traumatic brain**

**injury (TBI) was only recently designated as an SSDI category, so if
your survivor was turned down in the past, CALL AGAIN!**

To qualify for SSI: your survivor's income and resources must be
limited.

New SSDI disability and review determination process.

Designed to shorten decision times, starting in 2006 a new process built
upon electronic claims was phased in by region. Favorable decisions are
to be made within 20 days after the complete claim is received. The
process includes a new national network of experts "to enhance the
expertise needed to make accurate and timely decisions." **If benefits are
denied, appeal!** A new review process starts with a Federal Reviewing
Official who reviews state agency determinations, **if you request it**. If
you disagree with the decision made by this official, you still retain the
right to a hearing with an Administrative Law Judge. A Decision Review
Board also reviews and corrects decisional errors (Social Security
Online).

If you don't live in a region using the new process, the first step in
making an appeal is simply to apply for "reconsideration" with more
evidence from more doctors and more reports. Why reapply? About 2/3
of all applicants are denied benefits the first time and about 90% of all
first appeals are denied. But about 70% of those who persevere
ultimately receive their benefits (Abrams, 1999). *So keep trying and fight
for them!*

Do we need to hire an attorney? When? What is the cost?

If your survivor is denied benefits, yes. Contact an attorney as soon as
possible. The sooner the attorney can prepare, analyze, and gather
evidence, the better the chances of winning. Legal cases are generally
viewed with more respect — people who are represented are much more
successful than those who are not (Abrams, 1999). An attorney is also
invaluable when dealing with doctors and with the presiding judge. Legal
fees are usually 25% of past-due benefits and contingency-based (if the
case is lost, no fee is paid, except out-of-pocket copying, etc.).

Personal experience. *Thanks to my attorney, I finally received SSDI benefits — 12 years after my injury. It took that long mostly because of two factors: ignorance (mine and others) about how the system works — for example, denials are typical — and head injury wasn't considered a disability at the time of my injury.*

Supplemental Security Income (SSI)

Your loved one qualifies for this cash assistance program if he has few resources, is age 65 or older, blind, or disabled. Nationwide, the cash assistance rates increased from $674 in 2009 for an individual and from $1011 for a couple, with further yearly increases anticipated. The amount of benefit depends upon where he lives — some states supplement the basic amount (Social Security Online).

Resources, not including ownership of auto or home and attached land, must not exceed $2000 for single people or $3000 for couples. Any retirement accounts must be exhausted and all work income affects SSI benefits.

To determine benefit amount, monies *not* counted include the first $20 of most income received in a month, the first $65 earned from employment and half the amount over $65, home energy assistance, food stamps, and food and clothing received from non-profits (Social Security Online).

Social Security Work Incentives

Employment affects both SSDI and SSI benefits in several ways.

Trial Work Period — SSDI

To test work readiness, a disabled person is allowed a Trial Work Period (TWP) of a total of nine consecutive or interrupted "Trial Work Months" within a 60-month period. During this time, he can earn any amount and still receive full SSDI benefits.

A "Trial Work Month" allows a wage or self-employed earnings of up to $640 in 2007 and up to $670 in 2008 or working more than 80 self-employed hours in a month. This TWP threshold increased about $20-30 per month every year in the last few years. An "Extended Period of

Eligibility" (EPE) of 36 months follows the TWP during which the disabled worker can still receive benefits for any month his earnings are not "substantial" i.e. not more than $970 in 2009. Benefits may be reinstated without application. After this EPE period, if a job is lost, he needs to reapply for benefits (Social Security Online).

Substantial Gainful Activity (SGA) — SSDI & SSI
Substantial Gainful Activity is work that earns more than $970 per month in 2009. This increased during each of the last two years. Blind recipients can earn about $650 more per month. After your survivor completes nine trial work months (TWP), the "Substantial Gainful Activity" (SGA) level determines whether his earnings replace cash benefits. If his earnings fall below the SGA level, full cash benefits "generally continue." This limit increases to reflect greater living costs and applies to those not in a TWP.

If earnings are higher than the SGA level, cash benefits stop but medical benefits continue. If your survivor finds himself unable to continue working after five years above the SGA level, he needs to reapply. If employed less than five years, there is no need to reapply (Social Security Online).

Unsuccessful Work Attempt (SSDI & SSI)
If your survivor stopped or reduced his effort to do "substantial" work or self-employment to below the SGA level after six months or less because of his impairment or the loss of special conditions that allowed him to work, this is an Unsuccessful Work Attempt. For SSDI, earnings during this period are not counted toward SGA decisions except during the EPE. For SSI, these attempts are only considered at the time he first files a claim for benefits. (Social Security Online)

Impairment-Related Work Expenses (IRWE) — SSDI & SSI
Certain work-related items or services are deducted from gross SSDI earnings to determine if your survivor is earning SGA amounts or from SSI "earned income" without a decrease in benefits. Eligible deductions include those:
- That enable him to work.
- Required because of his disabling condition.

- That he paid the cost of and that are not reimbursed by another source.
- For which the cost is "reasonable" or standard in your community.
- For which he paid during a month that he worked.

    Examples include (Social Security Online):
- Attendant care services, which can include family members.
- Transportation costs, modifications to your vehicle or driver/taxi costs.
- Wheelchairs or special equipment, all impairment-related work-assistive devices, services, or systems, including service animals.
- Prostheses.
- Residential modifications.
- Regularly prescribed medical treatment to control your survivor's disabling condition.
- Medical supplies.
- Costs of a service animal.

SSI: Work and School Incentives

Student Earned Income Exclusion
This is good news for students! If your survivor is under age 22 and regularly attends school, he can earn $1640 in one month in 2009 (an increase of 5.8% from 2008) or $6600 in 2009 without affecting either eligibility or benefits. "Regularly attends" means he attends at least eight hours a week in college or at least 12 hours a week in a training course to prepare him for employment. He also may qualify if he is homebound due to disability (Social Security Online).

SSI Work Incentives
The amount of SSI payments is based upon the amount of any other income. When other monies increase, SSI decreases. If your survivor works, the first $65 ($85 if no other income) of earnings in a month are disregarded. After that, for every $2 that he earns, $1 is deducted from the SSI payment. If the job is lost, benefits revert to the original amount.

If there is a cut in pay, benefits increase. There is no Trial Work Period (TWP) (Social Security Online).

Pilot Projects
To increase employment, several pilot projects are under way in different states that could assist your survivor, including "Youth Transition Demonstrations." "National Benefit Offset" studies allow SSDI beneficiaries to work without total loss of benefits. Contact Social Security to learn if your state is involved or if other such pilot projects are under development.

The SSI Plan to Achieve Self-Support (PASS)

This is my favorite Social Security program! If he's eligible for SSI and has other income or resources besides what's needed for living expenses, your survivor qualifies. He can "set aside" this other income to obtain retraining or go to school to reach a work goal or start a business. SSI PASS really works! See *Brain Injury Rewiring for Survivors* for more information.

Subsidized Housing through HUD Section 8

If your survivor's income is reduced — whether or not he qualifies for SSI — encourage him to apply for the federal housing program called Section 8. Just as with SSDI, time is money — the sooner the process is begun, the sooner benefits begin. The usual waiting list time is 5 years.

Personal experience. As with other aspects of the rewiring process, securing post-injury housing is filled with shorts, frayed wires, and often what feels like dropped connections. However, good people appear to connect us — if we reach out. Encourage him to persist!

Obtain Retraining/Education

Attend school after injury. Why? How? What kind?
Your survivor will no doubt ask these questions. Whether returning to original fields or those closely allied but less demanding, if he improves his skills, he increases his marketability. For example, a degreed

professional may earn an assistant certificate at a community college to continue in the same line of work, but at a lower level of responsibility.

Obtain cognitive retraining.

Research has shown that improving cognitive skills positively affects both physical damage from and the emotional reaction to survivors' injury and is associated with enhanced community reentry. In other words, survivors who

> Let me tell you the secret that has led me to my goal. My strength lies in my tenacity.
> — Louis Pasteur

participate in cognitive retraining increase their odds of attaining some kind of normalcy.

Other retraining/employment options.

If your survivor does not feel ready to return to his original career field and/or does not want to work at a lower level or part-time or on-call, there are still more options!

Vocational inventories are available at career counseling offices at colleges and other places. These explore his interests and preferred environments — past or current — and thus reveal many work fields to investigate. Many young survivors are still exploring their interests at the time of injury and older ones may rediscover previous loves.

Electronic Memory Devices for Job Success

Prosthetic memory devices are especially useful cognitive assistants. These electronic brains can help your survivor return to work. A computer program, the expert shell system, used for years by

> The sun shines not on us, but in us.
> — John Muir

government and business, provides a structure for work tasks.

Therapists can develop software to perform decision-making functions modeled after a work setting. This reduces complex work-related questions to simple questions that can be answered by anyone. The therapist trains your survivor to use the "expert shell system" to do the job. Electronic brains to the rescue! People are still vital to the success of the expert shell in these ways: examining work tasks to be completed, reducing these jobs to a set of rules, entering this data into the shell system, consulting with the survivor concerning specific situations, training and monitoring him in use of the software, and modifying the rule structure until your survivor can meet accuracy standards (Parente & Parente, 1991).

When is the expert shell system not recommended?

For tasks that are too simple or too complex or that require human judgment and/or abstraction, a simple computer program may work better. But it is clear that advantages of the expert shell system far outweigh disadvantages. Thus, it can be a big win for employers, insurance companies, and most of all, for your survivor.

Getting Fired/Not Hired

Survivor or able-bodied, getting fired feels more or less the same every time — awful.

Fired and/or not getting hired.

If your survivor is fired from a job, urge him to consider possible reasons, which can be numerous. The post-injury survivor personality usually plays a part. Your survivor's propensity for directness may not be appreciated and his inability to

> I just wish they'd tell me I'm running out of straws before it's the last one.
> — Author

remember always poses problems. Maybe he tried too hard to fit in or to do the job, annoying less hard-working colleagues. Or maybe it wasn't his behavior — perhaps the work site was too busy or noisy — or any number of other "too" qualities! Although your survivor can ask why, his employer may be reluctant to give grounds, citing the American Disabilities Act (ADA) as responsible for employer fear of lawsuits. To help your survivor analyze what happened, stay positive and develop a plan for future jobs — use the SAFER plan.

Knowing why your survivor was not hired is also important. It's helpful for you or a counselor to team with him to assess his application and interview skills, again using the SAFER plan.

Self-Employment

This avenue can work for some survivors. Be sure to note the caveats and disadvantages in *Brain Injury Rewiring for Survivors*, so you can help him decide if this is a viable path for him to explore. If it is, your guidance — and perhaps also your business expertise — will be needed to make it successful!

> Often we look so long at the closed door that we don't even see the one that has opened for us.
> — Patricia Neal

Handling Rejection

Although you and other loved ones cannot immediately convince your survivor that he is okay whether or not he's doing productive work, what you can do is ask him what you can do to help. Ask what he thinks isn't okay, help him make and prioritize his list, and help him seek resources to shorten his list.

> Never let the fear of striking out get in your way.
> — Babe Ruth

Give Up?

Some survivors just give up the search altogether. It may be temporary — to relax, recharge, refocus — or it may be permanent and involve living with other relatives, homelessness, institutional care (jail or hospital), or death.

> Work is a four-letter word.
> — Victoria Cotton (a survivor who gave up)

Despite loved ones' care and concern, some survivors simply are not ready for this last step — productive work. It is no one's fault; it just can't happen now — or maybe ever. The hurdle is very, very high for some and can be a lifetime job in and of itself.

The responsibility to clear this last hurdle needs to remain with your survivor. You can assist and support, but you can't obtain or keep employment for him — that's up to him. What you can do is help your survivor to believe he can rewire!

Personal experience. Unfortunately, during a very painful and seemingly endless trial as a live-in helper for another survivor, I learned that — despite my best efforts — some people may choose the "give-up" option. Perhaps it served to remind me that a vital factor in recovery is the will to improve — despite setbacks.

Persevere?

I asked my doctor — who I came to realize much later was also my friend — many times, "How many doors do I have to knock on?" I asked in person, on the phone, and in my head starting in January 1980 when I was lucky enough to find him. And he always said, "As many as it takes." Remembering this exchange can transform a "poor me" outburst into a challenge with a goal — exactly what survivors need for job search. These words inspired me to continue to write *Brain Injury Rewiring* for over 30 years and to keep looking for a teaching opportunity that would work for me.

Summary

- Work is one of life's essentials.
- Volunteering can be a win-win solution.
- Most survivors return to productive activity.
- Family members can help just by being productive in their own lives.
- Many factors influence return to productive activity.
- A variety of work and vocational service programs are available.
- Apply for government benefit programs as soon as possible.
- Appeal, appeal, appeal if benefits are denied.
- SSDI and SSI can provide additional work and school incentives.
- Encourage and help your survivor to obtain retraining and education.
- Use the SAFER plan if he's fired/not hired.

> I was taught that the way of progress is neither swift nor easy.
> — Marie Curie

Conclusion

Patience and faith is what the sea teaches...
patience and faith.

— Anne Morrow Lindbergh

Dear Loved Ones,

I hope that *Brain Injury Rewiring for Loved Ones* will be a lifeline for you as you help your survivor recover optimally from his brain injury. It is a tremendous, lifelong challenge, but you and he can do it!

See Resources to find what you need to help him on his journey and refer him to the Resources in *Brain Injury Rewiring for Survivors*, too, so he can help himself.

As in *Brain Injury Rewiring for Survivors*, I list the most important thoughts, ideas, and strategies here by chapter for a handy reference.

General Rewiring

- Ask him what he needs. If he says, "I don't know," suggest sleep, food, drink, exercise, change of scenery or activity or topic.

> Trust yourself. You know more than you think you do.
> — Benjamin Spock, MD

- Wait and give him time to process. Ask him when he's ready.
- Keep trying to help find activities that engage him.
- Encourage his participation in rehab and remind him of his goals.
- Role model and explore a wide range of interests with him.
- Help him create the habit of success at small tasks so he attempts other more complex projects.

- Don't patronize or criticize him.
- Invite him to join you in your activities. Accompany him to local brain-injury foundation meetings.
- Remember that what works today may not work tomorrow.
- Keep hope alive for the best outcome, but be prepared for problems or setbacks to prevent limiting his potential and to minimize despair.
- Establish with the help of professionals what is and is not possible to change. What he can change will dictate the best course of action and whether to compensate or substitute for a deficit.
- Surround him with stimulating and positive people.
- Create a healthy environment with natural light, plants, and pets.
- Ensure he spends time every day with Nature.
- Work with a therapist to devise a recovery program.
- Consider the interrelationship of all the parts of our brains — often resolving one problem significantly impacts other problems.

Spiritual

- Change your home environment to fit his needs now.
- Chart your hearts.
- Play the music that's best for each of your activities.

> Nothing happens unless first a dream.
> — Carl Sandburg

- To avoid distress, learn what sounds and noises overload his wires, then flee, fight, or negotiate.
- If escape isn't possible, remind him to drown out the offending noise with his choice of music.
- Help him to ground himself if he escaped the noise too late.
- If you profess a faith, first look to it for ways that heal.
- Perform music to gain even more benefits than listening.
- Join him in his pursuit of creative arts.

Cognitive

- Know that the brain grows new cells and forms new networks.
- One side of the brain can compensate for the other side.
- An interesting environment will spur new growth.

> Just fix my brain and I won't be crazy! (or dumb or lazy or inappropriate ...)
> — Carolyn E. Dolen

- Survivors keep improving as long as they work at it.
- Improvement in cognitive functioning leads to involvement and improvement in all other types of treatment.
- Make to-do lists with step-by-step plans and review them.
- Design short and easy projects with a measurable end product.
- Work word and number games together.
- Play special learner-friendly music or white noise.
- Play games for an enjoyable way to learn or practice a skill.
- Ask only one question at a time.
- Help him analyze his needs.
- Don't question what he tells you.
- Do ask, "How have you set yourself up to succeed?"
- Model appropriate behavior and pay attention to your choice of words.
- Use and encourage positive self-talk.

Emotional

- Understand that trauma reactions are like grief responses.
- Know that his behavior, not him, is at fault.
- Do not accept undesirable behavior.

> Grief can't be worked out if people don't talk about the person who has died.
> — William Pinsof

- Know that rebuilding self-esteem at this stage of life is similar to developing it in his first few years of life.
- Seek the help of a mental health professional when your survivor demonstrates depression, aggression, or suicidal behavior.

- Express condolence with a touch, a hug, or just silent companionship — there may be little need for words.
- Consider healing rituals and creating your own memorial rite for his change.
- Allow yourselves to grieve, too.
- Be alert for substance abuse and seek treatment if it's suspected.
- Help him find ways to cope before he blows his circuits.
- Help him avoid known sources of distress and/or help him exit these places fast.
- Suggest ways to fight back with sounds of his choosing.
- Be alert for self-mutilation and suicidal ideation/intent — seek timely treatment.
- Remind him to get active. Exercise is proven to relieve stress.
- Offer understanding and listen with your heart.
- Provide perspective and companionship.
- Offer verbal and non-verbal support.
- Provide opportunities for control and decision-making.
- Seek community-based enrichment resources.
- Provide opportunities to deal with his anger.
- Your family also suffers, so strongly consider psychotherapy.

Conventional Medicine

- Know warning signs for depression.
- Effective medications are available.
- Maintain social connections to reduce your own depression.
- Continue treatment with a therapist only if they like each other.
- Consider using EMDR and neurofeedback for his recovery.
- Explore the use of vision and balance therapy.
- Investigate recent techniques to regain use of a damaged limb.
- Find aquatic, hippotherapy, and animal-assisted therapy.
- Seek expressive arts (music, drama, art) therapy programs.
- Consider using personal therapeutic devices, such as a light box.

> If you trust Google more than your doctor, then maybe it's time to switch doctors.
> — Jadelr and Cristina Cordova

- Investigate orthotics to correct structural misalignments.
- Prepare paperwork and your survivor for medical appointments.
- Survivors need to be empowered to heal themselves.

Complementary and Alternative Medicine

- Prevention of disease is superior to treatment of disease.
- Every organism possesses an energy that lives throughout the system and must flow freely.

> There are many paths up the mountain.
> — Rabbi Marc Gellman

- Acupuncture can correct imbalances and alleviate pain.
- Addictions and depression respond well to acupuncture.
- Investigate energy and hands-on healing methods.
- Know that many different kinds of massage are beneficial.
- Explore naturopathy, homeopathy, and osteopathy.
- Chiropractic care effectively treats back, neck, and joint injuries.
- Other manipulative techniques, like cranial sacral, work, too.
- Imagery, hypnosis, meditation, and magnetic therapy can help.

Nutrition

- Discuss his nutritional chapter with him.
- Remind him that his "car" needs premium fuel to run well.
- Discuss with him how bad food choices slow his recovery.
- Help him to choose healthy carbohydrates and eat more produce.

> We are indeed much more than what we eat, but what we eat can nevertheless help us to be much more than we are.
> — Adelle Davis

- Buy and prepare healthy food and order it when you dine out.
- Help him find ways to treat substance dependencies.
- Encourage him to create a routine for refreshing sleep.

Physical

- Believe that exercise benefits survivors in a big way!
- Know that length of time since injury or activity is unimportant.

> Movement and the functioning of the brain are eminently connected.
> — Rick Rogers

- Understand that if it took three million steps to learn to walk, why would take any fewer to relearn to walk?
- Set him up to succeed before he starts.
- Encourage him to do physical activities he likes every day.
- Remind him to schedule his activities.
- Investigate programs to improve his movement.
- Explore accessible gardening and relaxation activities.
- Seek places that offer help with physical activity.

Social

- His social problems result from what he does, not who or what he is.
- He can learn new behaviors because brains are adaptable.
- If you expect certain behaviors, he needs to know exactly what to do.

> Treat people as if they were what they ought to be and you help them to become what they are capable of becoming.
> — J. Van Goethe

- Dysfunctional behaviors caused by cognitive impairments will improve with better mental function even years after injury.
- Not all social glitches result from his mistakes.
- Support whatever your survivor feels successful doing.
- Rewiring social skills is just another skill aspect of rehabilitation.
- Social interaction is essential to his recovery.
- Affirming and welcoming people and places do exist.
- "Keep knocking on doors" to find these people and places.
- Use SAFER to prepare for his social activities.
- Know that counseling helps families better manage their feelings.
- Reduce or eliminate stressors related to household tasks.
- Maximize capabilities of family members, including your survivor.

- Believe that post-injury marriage can succeed — with lots of work.
- Social support decreases stress and is vital for family functioning.
- Social Skills/Conversation Improvement Programs are effective.
- Programs and strategies can improve behavior and social skills.
- Follow social strategy do's and don'ts.

Vocational

- Work is one of life's essentials.
- Volunteering can be a win-win solution.
- Most survivors return to productive activity.

> Let me tell you the secret that has led me to my goal. My strength lies in my tenacity.
> — Louis Pasteur

- Family members can help just by being productive in their own lives.
- Many factors influence return to productive activity.
- A variety of work and vocational service programs are available.
- Apply for government benefit programs as soon as possible!
- Appeal, appeal, appeal if benefits are denied.
- SSDI and SSI provide work and school incentives.
- Encourage and help him to obtain retraining and education.
- Use SAFER if he's fired/not hired.

Resources

Organizations that can help with all phases of brain injury rewiring are listed first in this section. Following that, resources are arranged in the same order as the chapters.

Go to www.rewiring.org for up-to-date recovery information and resources that also include books and DVDs.

General and Disability Information

American Association of People with Disabilities (AAPD)
> The largest cross-disability member organization in the US. Offers many benefits.
> www.aapd.com, 800-840-8844

American Brain Tumor Association
> Promotes research and offers information and support.
> www.abta.org, 800-886-2282

American Stroke Association (a division of American Heart Association)
> Information & resources for both survivors and caregivers; free subscription to *Stroke Connection Magazine*. Links include a national network of local support groups.
> www.strokeassociation.org, 888-4-STROKE ((888-478-7653)

Brain Injury Association, USA
> Provides information, education, and support to survivors, loved ones, and professionals. Many state affiliates, local chapters and support groups.
> www.biausa.org, 800-444-6443

Brainline.org
> Information on preventing, treating, and living with traumatic brain injury; funded by the Defense and Veterans Brain Injury Center.
> www.brainline.org, 703-998-2020

Centre for Neuro Skills
> Offers information, resources, services, products, and rehab programs for TBI. Products include: cognitive software, one-handed keyboard, vision restoration therapy device. Its TBI Resource Guide is the largest on-line bookstore for TBI.
> www.neuroskills.com, 800-922-4994

Disability-Related Information and Resources: This federal website provides comprehensive information about programs, services, laws and benefits in nine areas that include education, employment, health, housing, technology, and transportation. Find state and local resources in all these areas using a map.
> www.disabilityinfo.gov, various phone numbers on website.

Disability Resources Monthly (DRM)
> Guide to Disability Resources on the Internet. Updated daily. Provides well-organized access to thousands of resources for independent living arranged by state and subdivided by topic.
> www.disabilityresources.org, contact information on website.

Epilepsy Foundation of America (EFA)
> Provides information, resources, advocacy, and links to local foundations.
> www.efa.org, 800-332-1000

Family Village: A Global Community of Disability-Related Resources
> User-friendly website that integrates information, adaptive products, technology, recreational activities, education.
> www.familyvillage.wisc.edu/

Healthfinder (US Dept. of Health & Human Services)
> General health information on over 1600 topics from trusted sources. Find services and information. Free health interactive tools.
> www.healthfinder.gov/

Lash & Associates Publishing/Training
Traumatic brain injury books, brain injury information, and resources.
www.lapublishing.com, 919-562-0015

National Health Information Center (NHIC)
A resource database and referral service to link you with organizations that can answer health questions.
www.health.gov/nhic (various phone numbers on the site)

National Institute of Neurological Disorders and Stroke (NINDS)
Information on disorders from A to Z, materials, research, resources.
www.ninds.nih.gov, 800-352-9424

National Rehabilitation Information Center (NARIC)
Offers an abundance of resources: employment, advocacy, benefits, financial assistance, education, technology, and more.
www.naric.com, 800-346-2742

New Horizons Un-Limited
More than 2500 international links to information, products, resources, guides, events, programs, reference library, news; includes technology, recreation, arts, education, employment.
www.new-horizons.org

Traumatic Brain Injury National Resource Center (NRCTBI)
Helpful information for survivors and loved ones that includes personalized responses to questions, articles, products, conferences, links, FAQs.
www.neuro.pmr.vcu.edu

United Cerebral Palsy (UCP)
Information and resources in many areas, including products and services; research and advocacy for people with all disabilities.
www.ucp.org, 800-872-5827

United Spinal Association (USA)
Over 1900 sources of information/products on its usatechguide.org site; offers links, services.
www.unitedspinal.org, 800-404-2898

Family/Loved Ones

Family Caregiver Alliance (FCA)
> National Center on Caregiving. Education, information, services, research, and advocacy for caregivers; state-by-state guide of available help from all sources.
> www.caregiver.org, 800-445-8106

National Family Caregivers Association.
> Educates, supports, empowers, and advocates for all caregivers. Home of statewide Caregiving Community Action Network.
> www.nfcacares.org, 800-896-3650

Southern Caregiver Resource Center (CRC)
> Information, referral, support groups, counseling, consultation, and conferences for San Diego area; Link to 11 statewide CRCs. Also call Area Agencies on Aging in US or dial 211.
> www.caregivercenter.org, 800-827-1008

Books

Zasler ND, Katz D, & Zafonte R (eds). (2007). *Brain Injury Medicine: Principles and Practice*. Demos Publishers. 2007.

Equipment/Products/Technology Information

AbleData
> Provides database of unbiased information about assistive technology products and rehabilitation equipment available worldwide. Helps locate companies that sell these products.
> www.abledata.com, 800-227-0216

AbleLink Technologies
> Offers products to help with cognitive impairments.
> www.ablelinktech.com

RESNA
> Offers information about assistive technology and tries to connect visitors with experts in their area.
> www.resna.org, 703-524-6686

Alliance for Technology Access
> Network of community-based resource centers. Offers free
> service to locate and receive information on assistive technology
> products to promote independence.
> www.ataccess.org, 707-778-3011

Bruce Medical Supply
> General health and medical supplies, some sale items reduced to
> 35%. Free catalog.
> www.brucemedical.com, 800-225-8446

Center for Assistive Technology (CAT)
> Helps people find, select, and learn to use assistive technology
> devices and equipment for essential everyday needs: mobility,
> hearing, speech, and recreation as well as computer, vehicle, and
> home modifications.
> www.cat.pitt.edu, 412-647-1310

Center for Rehabilitation Technologies (CRT)
> Offers programs to assist people with physical disabilities to
> increase their independence
> www.helenhayeshospital.org/special_services/crt.htm,
> 888-70-REHAB (888-707-3422)

Disability Product postcards
> Information about catalogs and many products/equipment in a
> free monthly packet.
> www.blvd.com/dpp.htm

Cognitive

National Aphasia Association
> Provides information, support and advocacy; sells printed
> materials. Lists professionals, support groups, and treatment
> centers by state.
> www.aphasia.org, 800-922-4622

National Center for Learning Disabilities
> Offers information and resources for parents, educators, and
> students.
> www.ncld.org, 888-575-7373

HANDLE Institute (Holistic Approach to Neurodevelopment and
   Learning Efficiency)
   Provides clinical services and community information to identify
   and treat most neurodevelopmental disorders. Lists numerous
   regional practitioners.
   www.handle.org, 206-204-6000

Computer Equipment and Software; Internet Games/Exercises

Parrot Software
   Software for communication, memory, attention, speech, and
   cognitive rehabilitation. Offers free trial of internet programs.
   www.parrotsoftware.com, 800-727-7681

HAPPYneuron Brain Fitness
   Offers membership with unlimited and ever-changing games for
   $10/month.
   www.happy-neuron.com, various phone numbers on website.

Thinks.com
   Puzzles & Games: Sudoku, Crosswords, Chess, Checkers &
   more.
   www.thinks.com

Luminosity
   Brain training games.
   www.lumosity.com

Emotional

Depression and Bipolar Support Alliance (DBSA)
   Information, resources, support, products.
   www.dbsalliance.org, 800-826-3632
   Crisis line number: 800-273-TALK (800-273-8255)

Grief Recovery Online (GROWW)
   Chat rooms, message boards, news and information, resource
   lists, and support groups for all bereaved people.
   www.groww.org

Grief Recovery Helpline
> Answers questions about loss and recovery.
> www.ggcoa.org/r-hl-grief-recovery-helpline.htm, 800-445-4808

Mental Health America (MHA)
> Crisis help and information about disorders, treatments,
> medication, finding a therapist.
> www.nmha.org, 800-969-6642

National Alliance on Mental Illness (NAMI)
> Largest grassroots organization for those who are ill and their
> families, with affiliates in every state and many communities,
> offers information, education, support, advocacy, and helpline.
> www.nami.org, 800-950-NAMI (800-950-6264)

National Clearinghouse for Alcohol and Drug Information (NCADI)
> One-stop resource for information about substance abuse
> prevention and addiction treatment. Confer with information
> specialist, obtain referrals and order publications.
> www.ncadi.samhsa.gov, 800-729-6686

National Institute on Drug Abuse (NIDA)
> Information, materials, and resources for students and young
> adults, parents and teachers, and health professionals.
> www.nida.nih.gov, 301-443-1124

National Institutes of Mental Health (NIMH)
> Research focused on understanding, treating, and preventing
> mental disorders and promoting mental health.
> www.nimh.nih.gov, 866-615-6464

Substance Abuse and Mental Health Services Administration
(SAMHSA)
> Information about national programs, resources, services, and
> finding help.
> www.samhsa.gov, 800-662-HELP (800-662-4357)

Suicide Awareness Voices of Education (SAVE)
> Information, resources, and products for depression and suicide.
> www.save.org, National Suicide Prevention Lifeline 800-273
> TALK (800-273-8255), other numbers on website.

Traditional Medical

General Information

Centers for Disease Control and Prevention (CDC)
> Credible information on all known conditions and diseases as well as healthy living and environmental health topics.
> www.cdc.gov, 800-CDC-INFO (800-232-4636)

Mayo Clinic
> Medical services, information on symptoms, diseases and conditions, drugs and supplements, and healthy living. Includes "Ask a specialist" feature, newsletter.
> www.mayoclinic.com

Medscape
> Provides the latest medical news and access to journal articles on lots of topics.
> www.medscape.com

WebMD
> Features include pill identifier, symptom checker, find doctors and hospitals, medical news, health A to Z, nutritional information, blogs.
> www.webmd.com

Specific Conditions/Treatments

American Tinnitis Association (ATA)
> Information, answers to questions, advocacy, resources, newsletter, products, lists professionals and support groups in your area.
> www.ata.org, 800-634-8978

Animal-Human Connection
> Many programs and resources, including service animal and pet therapy, links, products.
> www.deltasociety.org, 425-679-5500

Canine Companions for Independence
> Trained assistance dogs free of charge.
> www.cci.org, 800-572-BARK (800-572-2275)

Eye Movement and Desensitization and Reprocessing (EMDR) Institute
Technique found to be highly effective for trauma. Includes
information, FAQs, references, locating clinicians.
www.emdr.com, 831-761-1040

Mobility Opportunities Via Education/Experience (MOVE) International
A worldwide program to help people gain independence and
improve mobility; model sites, research, products, FAQs, events.
www.move-international.org, 800-397-MOVE (800-397-6683)

Parents Active for Vision Education (PAVE)
Information, resources, products, blogs, referrals about visual
issues.
www.pavevision.org, 800-728-3988

Vestibular Disorders Association (VEDA)
Information, medical help, publications, products.
www.vestibular.org, 800-837-8428

Products, Devices

Cranial Electrical Stimulation Units (CES) and other healing light and
sound devices.
www.dynamind.com, 888-396-2646
www.sotainstruments.com, 800-224-0242

Light Therapy: many sources of light boxes available online.

Muscle Stimulation/Pain Management Units, including TENS: many
sites listed online.

Stroke Recovery Systems
Rehabilitation device to regain lost limb functionality.
www.neuromove.com, 800-845-1771

Complementary Medicine Resources

General Information

National Center for Complementary and Alternative Medicine
(NCCAM)
Offers research-based information on A to Z treatments and
conditions, FAQs, live online and phone help.
www.nccam.nih.gov, 888-644-6226

Health World Online
> Provides trustworthy information on wellness, healthy living, alternative therapies, body-mind-spirit health; finding practitioners.
> www.healthy.net

Specific Treatments

American Association of Acupuncture & Oriental Medicine (AAAOM)
> Consumer portion offers information, history, referrals, links.
> www.aaaomonline.org, 866-455-7999

American Chiropractic Association
> Patient section offers information, history, links, referrals, FAQs.
> www.amerchiro.org

American Massage Therapy Association
> Consumer section offers information, resources, links, find therapist, FAQs.
> www.amtamassage.org, 877-905-2700

American Osteopathic Association (AOA)
> Holistic medicine; information, links, resources, FAQs.
> www.osteopathic.org; 800-621-1773

American Society of Clinical Hypnosis
> Public site explains uses, myths, offers links, referrals, resources.
> www.asch.net, 630-980-4740

Energy Healing: These methods focus and amplify your life force (Chi) to help your body to naturally heal itself; sites offer history, information, practitioners, resources, blog.
> www.quantumtouch.com, 888-424-0041
> www.reiki.com

Feldenkrais Method of Somatic Education:
> Offers information, resources, FAQs, publications.
> www.feldenkrais.com, 800-775-2118

Trager Approach
> History, information, find practitioner, articles.
> www.trager.com

World Wide Online Meditation Center|
> Offers information, instruction on many techniques, resources, books, products, FAQs.
> www.meditationcenter.com

Nutrition

General Information

Center for Science in the Public Interest (CSPI)
> Nutrition and health, public safety, and sound science; "Nutrition Action" is largest circulation health newsletter in North America.
> www.cspinet.org, 202-332-9110

Harvard School of Public Health, Dept. of Nutrition
> Healthy eating guidelines and tips, recipes, FAQs, dispels myths.
> www.hsph.harvard.edu/nutritionsource

Mayo Clinic Nutrition and Healthy Eating
> Information about healthy eating and cooking, free newsletter.
> www.mayoclinic.com/health/nutrition-and-healthy-eating/MY00431

Queensland nutrition website
> Healthy eating, activity, and food safety tips, news, and resources.
> www.health.qld.gov.au/healthieryou/food

US Dept. of Agriculture
> Lots of info, guidelines, helps to plan/track health and activity to manage weight/eating, resources, links.
> www.mypyramid.gov, 888-7-PYRAMID (888-779-7264)

Also see General Information under Traditional Medical

Physical

General Fitness/Health Information

MyStart!
> Free American Heart Association (AHA) online tool to help
> people make positive lifestyle changes through physical activity
> and better eating.
> www.americanheart.org/presenter.jhtml?identifier=3053103

Disability-Related Fitness/Sports/Recreation

Blaze Sports
> Provides sports training, competitions, summer camps, and other
> recreational opportunities to youth and adults with disabilities;
> current calendar, magazine; memberships available.
> www.blazesports.org, 770-850-8199

Disabled Sports USA
> Nationwide network of community-based chapters that offers
> sports and recreational programs; magazine, equipment
> resources.
> www.dsusa.org, 301-217-0960

Disabled Sports USA Far West
> Offers special events, plus 200+ program days, links, newsletter.
> www.dsusafw.org, 916-722-6447

Disaboom
> An interactive online disability community for people with
> disabilities and their loved ones; offers health-lifestyle
> information, news, groups, blogs.
> www.disaboom.com

National Center on Physical Activity and Disability (NCPAD)
> Comprehensive information on many disabilities/conditions,
> including all aspects of fitness programs; organized by state and
> country, suppliers, references, resources, videos, research;
> nutrition; newsletter; search mechanism; free information
> service. Free "virtual trainer" tips sent by email.
> www.ncpad.org, 800-900-8086

National Sports Center for the Disabled
>   Offers adaptive recreation clinics and programs in over 20 sports throughout the US, including competitive skiing.
>   www.nscd.org, 970-726-1540

Re-Creative Resources, Inc.
>   "Recreating mind, body and spirit" website that lists hundreds of products and providers; links, resources; go to Resources/Links, then Programming for adaptive equipment, leisure activities, crafts, music.
>   www.recreativeresources.com, 732-340-1210

Specific Activities/Sports/Populations

Active Network
>   nationwide listing of events in all sports, registration, training logs, nutrition, training and fitness tips, resources, race results, blogs.
>   www.active.com

Our Ocean Dreams
>   Aquatic experiences; learn to dive anywhere there's water, nationwide network of divers; online certification courses.
>   www.ouroceandreams.com, 727-578-3095

Extremity Games
>   Yearly sports competition for those with limb loss or difference; events include Moto-X, skateboarding, rock climbing, wakeboarding, kayaking, mountain biking, martial arts; blog.
>   www.extremitygames.com, 586-556-1761

Holden Arboretum, Accessible Gardening/Horticulture Therapy
>   programs, classes, activities, tours, resources.
>   www.holdenarb.org, 440-946-4000

Hippotherapy (rehabilitative horseback riding), horticulture therapy;
>   supported employment; attractions include aquarium, rainforest.
>   www.moodygardens.com/Hope_Therapy, 800-582-4673

National Center for Equine Facilitated Therapy (CEFT)
>   Offers programs, activities, therapeutic riding.
>   www.nceft.org, 650-851-2271

Wheelchair Sports, Recreation & Accessible Travel
> Lists 39 web sites that offer a variety of active programs for those with disabilities; links/resources.
> www.usatechguide.org

Equipment (listed by company)

Abilitations
> Specialized equipment for physical and mental development through movement. Products, articles, activity guides.
> www.abilitations.com, 800-850-8602

Access to Recreation, Inc.
> Wide range of indoor and outdoor adaptive equipment and products.
> www.accesstr.com, 800-634-4351

Achievable Concepts
> Australian company selling adapted recreation and sporting equipment products worldwide.
> www.achievableconcepts.com.au

FlagHouse
> A global supplier of over 20,000 physical education, recreation, health care products. Free catalog.
> www.flaghouse.com, 800-793-7900

S&S Worldwide
> Educational, rehab, and therapy products, games and activities. Free catalog.
> www.ssww.com, 800-288-9941

For sport-specific equipment, videos, journals, and books, go to Resources at www.rewiring.org

Social

Brain and Spinal Cord Injury Information and Support Groups
> blog, video library, resources.
> www.brainandspinalcord.org, 800-800-0640

Chat Rooms for survivors
> www.braininjurychat.org
> www.tbichat.org

Chat Rooms for survivors and loved ones, message boards, member
> pages
> www.tbihome.org

Vocational/Community Reentry

Education

Higher Education/Training for People with Disabilities (HEATH)
> Information, including financial assistance, for students with
> disabilities who seek post-secondary education and/or training.
> www.heath.gwu.edu

Employment

Job Accommodation Network (JAN)
> Free consultation, information, and technical support to job
> seekers and employers about opportunities, training, and rights.
> www.jan.wvu.edu, 800-526-7234

Office of Disability Employment Policy (ODEP)
> Information on employment supports; sites for veterans; links;
> resources.
> www.dol.gov/odep, 866-ODEP-DOL (866-633-7365)

Ticket to Work Program:
> For Social Security recipients. Obtain vocational rehabilitation
> services through your state agency and explore work options
> without losing benefits in this federal program. Employment
> regulations, supports, and work incentives; locate forms and
> publications.
> www.socialsecurity.gov/work, 800-772-1213

Traumatic Brain Injury National Resource Center
> Employment resources.
> www.neuro.pmr.vcu.edu/LINKS/employ.htm

Veterans' Employment and Training Service (VETS)
> Recovery & Employment Assistance Lifelines program
> (REALifelines) designed to provide a seamless, personalized
> assistance network for returning injured and wounded service
> members.
> www.dol.gov/vets, 866-4-USA-DOL (866-487-2365)

Financial/Legal

David L. Goldin, APC
> Articles, news, links, free consultation for survivors/loved ones;
> member of San Diego BIF.
> www.brain-injuries-law.com, 866-HEADLAW (866-432-3529)

Equal Employment Opportunities Commission (EEOC)
> General advice about ADA disability claims; how to file; locate
> local office.
> www.eeoc.gov, 800-669-4000

National Insurance Consumer Helpline
> Consumer support for questions and problems relating to
> insurance.
> www.cancerandcareers.org/resources/one?resource_id=56278,
> 800-942-4242

Renter Assistance: Call your state franchise tax board or Volunteer
Income Tax Assistance (see below) for application information.

Social Security Administration (SSA)
> Federal source to learn about, apply, and appeal for SSDI
> (disability) and SSI; locate forms and publications.
> www.ssa.gov, 800-772-1213

Veterans' Administration Benefits
> Information about education, rehabilitation, benefits, FAQs,
> finding facilities, links; apply online.
> www.vba.va.gov/VBA, 800-827-1000

Volunteer Income Tax Assistance
> IRS-sponsored program with volunteers to provide free tax
> preparation assistance to low income, disabled, and/or military
> filers.
> www.vita-volunteers.org

Housing/Medical

HUD-Federal Housing Authority (HA)
> Answers to questions about housing choice vouchers (Section 8), Self Sufficiency Program.
> www.hud.gov/renting, numerous 800 numbers on website

Medicare
> Medicare and Medicaid coverage, prescription plans; apply, appeal; ask questions.
> www.medicare.gov, 800-MEDICARE (800-633-4227)

Rural Information Center
> For those who live in rural areas; information about education, funding sources, health, and starting a business.
> ric.nal.usda.gov, 800-633-7701

Vocational Rehabilitation

Non-Vets: Search online by for your state agency, look under state listings in local phone book (it may be called Agency, Department, Division, or Office), or go to www.socialsecurity.gov/work, 800-772-1213, for "Ticket To Work" information

Veterans with service-connected disabilities: Vocational Rehabilitation and Employment Service (VR&E) provides evaluation, counseling, assistance, and training for vets to prepare for, find, and keep suitable jobs; site lists resources, links, how to apply www.vba.va.gov/bln/vre

References

Chapter Three: Brain Construction and Wiring

Askenasy, J.J., & Rahmani, L. (1987). Neuropsycho-social rehabilitation of head injury. *American Journal of Physical Medicine, 66*(6), 315-327.

Bach-y-Rita, P. (1981). Brain plasticity as a basis of the development of rehabilitation procedures for hemiplegia. *Scandinavian Journal of Rehabilitation Medicine, 13*:73-83.

Bach-y-Rita, P. (1981). Central nervous system lesions: Sprouting and unmasking in rehabilitation. *Archives of Physical Medicine and Rehabilitation, 62*:413-417.

Block, S. (1987). Psychotherapy of the individual with brain injury. *Brain Injury, 1*(2):203-206.

Bond, M.R. & Brooks, D.N. (1976). Understanding the process of recovery as a basis for the investigation of rehabilitation for the brain injured. *Scandinavian Journal of Rehabilitation Medicine, 8*:127-133.

Bray, L.J., Carlson, F. Humphrey, R., Mastrelli, J., & Valso, A. (1987). Physical rehabilitation. In Ylvisaker, M. & Gobble, E. (eds.). *Community re-entry for head injured adults*. Boston: College Hill.

Cobble, N.D., Bontke, C.F., Brandstater, M.E., & Horn, L.J. (1991). Rehabilitation in brain disorders: Three intervention strategies. *Archives of Physical Medicine and Rehabilitation, 72*:S324-S331.

Cohadon, F., Richter, E., Reglade, C., & Dartigues, J.F. (1988). Recovery of motor function after severe traumatic coma. *Scandinavian Journal of Rehabilitation Medicine. Supplement, 17*:75-85.

Edelstein, B.A., & Couture, E.T. (1984). *Behavioral assessment and rehabilitation of the traumatically brain-damaged*. New York: Plenum Press.

Frazee, John. (1997). *Bottom line personal. 18*(17). Brain damage from strokes can be prevented.

Goldberg, S. (1979). *Clinical neuroanatomy made ridiculously simple*. Miami: Medmaster, Inc.

Golden, C.J. (1978). Diagnosis and rehabilitation in clinical neuropsychology. Chicago: Charles C Thomas.

Gray, H.G. (1977). Anatomy, descriptive and surgical. (Gray's Anatomy: The Classic Collector's Edition). New York: Bounty Books.

Hackler, E & Tobis, J.S. (1983). Reintegration into the community. In Rosenthal, M., Griffith, E.R., Bond, M.R., Miller, J.D. (eds.). *Rehabilitation of the head-injured adult*. Philadelphia: F.A. Davis.

Haffey, W.J. & Lewis, F.D. (1989). Rehabilitation outcomes following traumatic brain injury. *Physical Medicine and Rehabilitation: State of the Art Reviews, 3*(1):203-218.

Hook, O. (1988). Head injury. *Scandinavian Journal of Rehabilitation Medicine. Supplement, 17*:65-74.

Howieson, D. & Lezak, M. (1992). The neuropsychological evaluation. In Yudofsky, S. & Hales, R. (eds.). *Textbook of neuropsychiatry*. Washington, D.C.: The American Psychiatric Press.

Iowa Healthbook: Brain injury — A Guide for families and friends. (1997). University of Iowa. Librarian The Virtual Hospital.@vh.org. 4/28/97

Kreutzer, J.S., Leininger, B.E., Harris, J.A. (1990). The evolving role of neuropsychology in community integration. In Kreutzer, J. & Wehman, P. (eds.). *Community integration following traumatic brain injury*. Baltimore: Brookes Publishing.

Lehr, R.P. (1997). *Brain function*. Southern Illinois University.

Manzi, D.B., & Weaver, P.A. (1987). *Head injury: The acute care phase*. New York: Slack.

Miller, L. (1993). *Psychotherapy of the brain-injured patient: Reclaiming the shattered self*. New York: Norton.

Minteer-Convery, M.A. (1985). Head injury. *Annual Review of Rehabilitation*, *4*:215-239.

Najenson, T., Mendelson, L., Schechter, I., David, C., Mintz, N., & Groswasser, Z. (1974). Rehabilitation after severe head injury. *Scandinavian Journal of Rehabilitation Medicine*, *6*:5-14.

Namerov, N.S. (1987). Cognitive and behavioral aspects of brain-injury rehabilitation. *Neurologic Clinics*, *5*(4):569-583.

Perry, J. (1983). Rehabilitation of the neurologically disabled patient: Principles, practice, and scientific basis. *Journal of Neurosurgery*, *58*:799-816.

Prigatano, G.P., Fordyce, D.J., Zuiner, H.K., Roueche, J.R., Pepping, M., & Wood, B.C. (1984). Neurological rehabilitation after closed head injury in young adults. *Journal of Neurology, Neurosurgery, & Psychiatry*, *47*:505-513.

Rayport, S. (1992). Cellular and molecular biology of the neuron. In Yudofsky, S. & Hales, R. (eds.). *Textbook of neuropsychiatry*. Washington, D.C.: The American Psychiatric Press.

Restak, R. (1992). You and your brain. *Bottom Line*, *13*(4).

Richey, R. (1993). Is head injury contagious? *Head Injury Press (HIP)*, *115*:2-3.

Sbordone, R. (1987). A conceptual model of neuropsychologically-based cognitive rehabilitation. In Williams, J. M. & Long, C.J. (eds.). *The rehabilitation of cognitive disabilities*. New York: Plenum Press.

Silver, J.M., Hales, R.E., & Yudofsky, S.C. (1992). Neuropsychiatric aspects of traumatic brain injury. In Yudofsky, S. & Hales, R. (eds.). *Textbook of neuropsychiatry*. Washington, D.C.: The American Psychiatric Press.

Stahl, S.M. (2000). *Essential psychopharmacology*. London, UK: Cambridge University Press.

Stein, D., Brailowsky, S., & Will, B. (1995), *Brain repair*. New York: Oxford University Press.

Stroke Recovery Systems. (2004). Specification and features: NM900. How does it work? www.neuromove.com/neuromovespecifications.html pp. 1-2, 9/21/2004

Szekeres, Ylvisaker, M., & Cohen. (1987). A framework for cognitive rehabilitation therapy. In Ylvisaker M. & Gobble E. (eds.). *Community re-entry for head injured adults*. Boston: College Hill.

Thomsen, I.V. (1984). Late outcomes of very severe blunt head trauma: A 10-15 year second follow-up. *Journal of Neurology, Neurosurgery, and Psychiatry*, *47*:260-268.

Timmons, M., Gasquoine, L., & Scibak, J.W. (1987). Functional changes with rehabilitation of very severe traumatic brain injury survivors. *Journal of Head Trauma Rehabilitation*, *2*(3):64-73.

TPN (The Perspectives Network, Inc.). 1997. dktaylor@tbi.org. 4/28/97.

Vogenthaler, D.R. (1987). Subject review. An overview of head injury: Its consequences and rehabilitation. *Brain Injury*, *1*(1):113-127.

Wachter, Fawber, & Scott. (1987). Vocational evaluation. In Ylvisaker M. & Gobble E. (eds.). *Community re-entry for head injured adults*. Boston: College Hill.

Zasler, N.D., Katz, D., & Zafonte, R. (eds). (2007). *Brain Injury Medicine: Principles and Practice*. Demos Publishers. 2007.

Chapter Four: Spiritual Rewiring

Barfield, C. (1998). A blend of faith: Native Americans here practice Catholicism while retaining much of their culture. It's called "syncretism." *The San Diego Union-Tribune, Current & Arts* section, Religion & Ethics, E-1, Friday, June 12, 1998.

Being Jewish: The hands-on supplement for Jewish Family Education, Passover 1998. (1998). David Epstein, publisher.

Campbell, D. (1998). *Bottom Line Personal*, January 15, 1998.

Campbell, D. (1997). *The Mozart effect: Tapping the power of music to heal the body, strengthen the mind, and unlock the creative spirit.* New York: Avon Books.

Carter, D. How music heals: Trends in the use of music and sound in healing, http: Holistic.com/essays/music01.htm.

Cool, L.C. (1997). Faith & healing. *American Health, 47.*

Craughwell, T. Ed. (1998). *Every eye beholds you: A world treasury of prayer.* New York:Book-of-the-Month Club. pp. xiv-xvii, 11, 13, 14, 17, 21-22, 171-172, 207-208, 225

Dharma Haven Home Page. http://dharma-haven.org/tibetan/meaning-of-om-mani-padme-hung.htm.

Grey, A. The history of art and healing, healing ourselves with art, how art heals: Mind-body physiology, art as a healing force. www.artashealing.org/ahfw10.htm.

Healthscope: (1997). Music to relax by. *American Health*, November 1997, p. 21

Metzger, B.M., Coogan, M.D. (eds.). (1993). *The Oxford companion to the Bible.* New York:Oxford University Press. pp. 27-28, 287-288, 499-500, 607-608, 668-669.

Phoenix & Arabeth (1999). Shamanic origin of the arts. www.zapcom.net/phoenix.arabeth/shaman.html.

Chapter Five: Cognitive Rewiring

Abdulla, S. (2001). Drill helps adult dyslexics. Brain imaging is hot on the trail of dyslexia. American Association for the Advancement of Science, San Francisco, February 2001, as reported in Science Update in www.nature.com/nsu/010222/010222-5.html

Askenasy, J. J., & Rahmani, L. (1987). Neuropsycho-social rehabilitation of head injury. *American Journal of Physical Medicine, 66*(6):315.

Ben-Yishay et al. (1987). Cited in Wachter, J., Fawber, H.L., & Scott, M.B. Vocational evaluation. In Ylvisaker M. & Gobble E. (eds.). *Community re-entry for head injured adults.* Boston: College Hill.

Deaton, A. (1991). Rehabilitating cognitive impairments through use of games. In Kreutzer, J. & Wehman, P. (eds.). *Community integration following traumatic brain injury.* Baltimore: Brookes Publishing.

Eriksson, P.S., Perfilieva, E., Björk-Eriksson, T., Alborn, A., Nordborg, C., Peterson, D.A. & Gage, F.H. (1998). Neurogenesis in the adult human hippocampus. *Nature Medicine, 4*(11):1313.

Hamm, R.J., Temple, M.D., O'Dell, D.M., Pike, B.R., & Lyeth, B.G. (1996). Exposure to environmental complexity promotes recovery of cognitive function after traumatic brain injury. *Journal of Neurotrauma, 13*(1):41-7.

Johnson, D.W. (1999). Antiaging strategies: for your body, for your mind. *Bottom Line Health. 13*(2):2.

Levin, W. (1991). Computer applications in cognitive rehabilitation. In Kreutzer, J. & Wehman, P. (eds.). *Community integration following traumatic brain injury.* Baltimore: Brookes Publishing.

Levine, B., Cabeza, R., McIntosh, A.R., Black, S.E., Grady, C.L., Stuss, D.T. (2002). Functional reorganization of memory after traumatic brain injury: A study with H2O positron emission tomography. *Journal Neurology Neurosurgery Psychiatry. 73*(2):111.

Najenson, T., Mendelson, L., Schechter, I., David, C., Mintz, N., & Groswasser, Z. (1974). Rehabilitation after severe head injury. *Scandinavian Journal of Rehab. Medicine, 6*:5.

Namerov, N.S. (1987). Cognitive and behavioral aspects of brain-injury rehabilitation. *Neurologic Clinics, 5*(4):569.

Parente, R. & Anderson-Parente, J.K. (1991). Retraining memory: Theory, evaluation, and applications. In Kreutzer, J. & Wehman, P. (eds.). *Community integration following traumatic brain injury.* Baltimore: Brookes Publishing.

Sbordone, R. (1991). Overcoming obstacles in cognitive rehabilitation of persons with severe traumatic brain injury. In Kreutzer, J. & Wehman, P. (eds.). *Community integration following traumatic brain injury.* Baltimore: Brookes Publishing.

Stein, D., Brailowsky, S. & Will, B. (1995). *Brain repair,* London, UK: Oxford University Press.

Vogenthaler, D.R. (1987). Subject review: An overview of head injury: Its consequences and rehabilitation. *Brain Injury, 1*(1):113.

Chapter Six: Emotional Rewiring

Addiction Science Network. (2000). The biological basis of addiction. www.addictionsciencenetwork.net/ASNbiological2.htm.

Archart-Treichel J. (2003). Data back relationship between serotonin binding, suicide attempts. *Psychiatric News, 38*(12):26-29.

Baser, C. (1997). Personal communication.

Bombardier, C.H., Edhe D., Kilmer, J. (1997). Readiness to change alcohol drinking habits after traumatic brain injury. *Archives Phy. Med Rehab, 78*(6):592-6.

Brown G.K., Ten Have T., Henriques G.R., Xie, S.X., Hollander, J.E., 7 Beck A.T. (2005). Cognitive therapy for the prevention of suicide attempts. *JAMA, 294*:563-570.

CAMH (Centre for Addiction and Mental Health), Univ. of Toronto. (2003). Link between serotonin and suicide found with new brain imaging methods. www.suicidereference library.com

Corrigan, J.D. (2003). Relationship between traumatic brain injury and substance abuse. Columbus, Ohio: Ohio Valley Center for Brain Injury Prevention and Rehabilitation.

Corrigan, J.D., Rust, E., & Lamb-Hart, G.L. (1995). The nature and extent of substance abuse problems in persons with traumatic brain injury. *Journal of Head Trauma Rehabilitation, 10*(3):29-46.

Corrigan, J.D., Bogner, J.A., Lamb-Hart, G.L., & Windisch, E. (1996). Effectiveness of a case management model for treatment of substance abuse following acquired brain injury. Columbus, Ohio: Ohio Valley Center for Head Injury Prevention and Rehabilitation.

Corrigan J.D., & Bogner L. (2007). Interventions to promote retention in substance abuse treatment. *Brain Injury, 21*(4):343-56.

Engstrom, G., Alling, C., Blennow, K., Regnell, G., & Traskman-Bendz. L. (1999). Reduced cerebrospinal HVA concentrations and HVA/5-HIAA ratios in suicide attemptors: Monamine metabolites in 120 suicide attemptors and 47 controls. *Eur Neuropsychopharmacol, 5*:399-405.

Falconer, J. Substance abuse and brain injury. *Brain Train.* www.brain-train.com/articles/substanc.html#SubstanceAbuse and Brain Injury.

Hendryx, P.M. (1989). Psychosocial changes perceived by closed head-injured adults and their families. *Archives of Physical Medicine and Rehabilitation, 70*:526-530.

Johnson, B., Rosenthal, N., Capece, J., Wiegand, F., Mao, L., Beyers, K., McKay, A., Ait-Daoud, N., Addolorado, G., Anton, R., Ciraulo, D., Kranzler, H., Mann, K., O'Malley, S., & Swift, R. (2008). Improvement of physical health and quality of life of alcohol-dependent individuals with topiramate treatment: US multisite randomized controlled trial. *Arch Intern Med., 168*(11):1188-1199.

Knowlton L. (1995). Scientists study serotonin markers for suicide prevention. *Psychiatric Times XII*(9).

Koob, G.F. (2006). Alcohol dependence: The importance of neurobiology to treatment. *Medscape Psychiatry & Mental Health, 11*(2).

Kreutzer, J., Marwitz, J.H., Witol, A.D. (1995). Interrelationships between crime, substance abuse, and aggressive behaviours among persons with traumatic brain injury. *Brain Injury, 9*(8):757-768.

Leon-Carrian, J., DeSerdio-Arias, M.L., Cabezas, F.M., Roldan, J.M., Domanquez-Morales, R., Maartan, J.M., Sanchez, M.A. (2001). Neurobehavioral and cognitive profile of traumatic brain injury patients at risk for depression and suicide. *Brain Injury, 15*(2):175-81.

Lovinger, D.P. (1999). The role of serotonin in alcohol's effects on the brain. *Current Separations, 18*(1):23-28).

Mameli-Engvall, M., Evrard, A., Pons, S., Maskos, U., Svensson, T., Changeux, J.P., Faure, P. (2006). Hierarchical control of dopamine neuron-firing patterns by nicotinic receptors. *Neuron.* June 15, 2006.

NIDA (National Institute on Drug Abuse). (2007). NIDA InfoFacts: Methamphetmine. NIH, March 2007.

NIDA. (2006). Research report: Methamphetamine abuse and addiction. *NIH Publication* #06-4210.

Oquendo, M.A., Friedman, J.H., Grunebaum, M.F., Burke, A., Silver, J.M., & Mann, J.J. (2004). Suicidal behavior and mild traumatic brain injury in major depression. *J Nerv Ment Dis, 192*(6):430-4.

Prigatano, G.P. (1995). 1994 Sheldon Berrol, MD, Senior lectureship: The problem of lost normality after brain injury. *Journal of Head Trauma Rehabilitation, 10*(3):87-95.

RTC: Research & Training Ctr. on Community Integration of Individuals with TBI. (2000). Consumer Report # 6: Coping with substance abuse after TBI. Mt. Sinai School of Med.

Rudd, M.D., Berman, A.L., Joiner, Jr. T.E., Nock, M.K., Silverman, M.M., Mandrusiak, M., Van Orden, K., & Witte, T. (2006). Warning signs for suicide: Theory, research, and clinical applications. *Suicide and Life-Threatening Behavior, 36*(3):255-262.

SAVE (Suicide Awareness Voices of Education). (2007). http://save.org/prevention.html. 3/20/2007.

Sbordone, R. (1987). A conceptual model of neuropsychologically-based cognitive rehabilitation. In Williams, J.M. & Long, C.J. (eds.). *The rehabilitation of cognitive disabilities*. New York: Plenum Press.

Sbordone, R. (1991). Overcoming obstacles in cognitive rehabilitation of persons with severe traumatic brain injury. In Kreutzer, J. & Wehman, P. (eds.). *Community integration following traumatic brain injury*. Baltimore: Brookes Publishing.

Simpson, G. & Tate, R. (2002). Suicidality after traumatic brain injury: Demographic, injury and clinical correlates. *Psychol Med., 32*(4):687-97.

Simpson, G. & Tate, R. (2005). Clinical features of suicide attempts after traumatic brain injury. *J Nerv Ment Dis, 193*(10):680-5.

Tanner, D.C. (1984). *Aphasia: The family's guide to the psychology of loss, grief, and adjustment*. Tulsa: Modern Education Corporation.

Taber's cyclopedic medical dictionary, 16th edition. (1989).

TBI consumer report #6: Coping with substance abuse after TBI. (2000). Research and Training Center, Mt. Sinai School of Medicine.

Teasdale, T.W. & Engberg, A.W. (2001). Suicide after stroke: A population study. *J Epidemiol Community Health, 55*:863-866.

Teasdale, T.W. & Engberg, A.W. (2001). Suicide after traumatic brain injury. *J Neurol Neurosurg Psychiatry, 71*(4):436-40.

Zasler, N.D. (1992). Neuromedical diagnosis and management of post-concussive disorders. *Physical Medicine and Rehabilitation: State of the Art Reviews, 6*(1):49-50, 61-62.

Chapter Seven: Conventional Medicine

Baser, C. (1998). Personal communication.

Bennington, K. (1997). Eye movement desensitization and reprocessing. Unpublished paper and personal communication.

Brink S. (2006). Depressed brain can be "primed." *LA Times*, F:1, F6. 8/7/06.

Centre for Neuro Skills. (1999). In the news… medication may prevent excitotoxic brain damage. *Inside View, 8.1*:4.

Centre for Neuro Skills. (2006). Long-term ibuprofen regimen after brain injury worsens cognition. *Experimental Neurology*, August 2006.

Dupler J. (1998). Neurofeedback as an alternative treatment for head injury. Unpublished; written for *Rewiring*.

Engberg, A. (1989). Vestibular stimulation after head injury: effect on reaction time and motor speech parameters. *Archives of Physical Medicine and Rehabilitation. 70*:893.

Ergh, T.C., Rapport, L.J., Coleman, R.D., & Hanks, R.A. (2002). Predictors of caregiver and family functioning following traumatic brain injury: Social support moderates caregiver distress. *J Head Trauma Rehabil, 17*(2):155-74.

Gardner, D. (1998). When to push pills: The role of medication treatment in TBI. *San Diego Brain Injury Press*, 7-92.

Gardner, D. (2007). Personal communication.

Thomas, C. (ed.). (1989). *Tabers cyclopedic medical dictionary.* Philadelphia: FA Davis. pp. 534, 949, 1764.

Lamotrigine in multi-handicapped therapy-resistant epileptic patients. (1998). *Clin. Drug. Invest, 16*(4):263.

Moldover, J.E., Goldberg, K.B., Prout,. M.F. (2004). Depression after traumatic brain injury: A review of evidence for clinical hetereogeneity. *Neuropsychol Rev., 14*(3):143-54.

Gianutsos, R., Ramsey, G., & Perlin, R. (1988). Rehabilitative optometric services for survivors of acquired brain injury. *Archives of Physical Medicine and Rehabilitation, 69*:573.

Gizzi, M. (1995). The efficacy of vestibular rehabilitation for patients with head trauma. *The Journal of Head Trauma Rehab. 10*(6):60.

Harvard Women's Health Watch. (1995). Light boxes. October 1995

Health Confidential. (1996). (Interview of George Brainerd) Light therapy to beat: Heart disease, insomnia, depression, and more. *Health Confidential,* 5. July 1996.

Hunter, A., Leuchter, A., Morgan, M., Cook, I. (2006). Changes in brain function (quantitative EEG cordance) during placebo lead-in and treatment outcomes in clinical trials for major depression. *Am J Psychiatry 163*:1426-1432.

Jorge, R.E., Robinson, R.G., Moser, D., Tateno, A., Crespo-Facorro, B., & Arndt, S. (2004). Major depression following traumatic brain injury. *Arch Gen Psychiatry, 61*(1):42-50.

Kimberly, T., Lewis, S., Auerbach, E., Dorsey, L., Lojovich, J., & Carey, J. (2004). Electrical stimulation driving functional improvements and cortical changes in subjects with stroke. *Experimental Brain Research, 154*(4):450-460.

Kirsch, D,. & Lerner, F. (1998). *Pain management: A practical guide for clinicians: The official textbook of the American Academy of Pain Management.* Chapter 55: Electro medicine: The Other Side of Physiology.

Kirsch, D.L. & Smith, R.B. (2000). The use of cranial electrotherapy in the management of chronic pain: A review. *NeuroRehabilitation, 14*(2):85-94.

Kirsch, D. (2002). *The science behind cranial electrotherapy stimulation.* 2nd edition. Medical Scope Publishing Corporation.

Klawansky, S., Yeung, A., Berkey, C., Shah, N., Phan, H., & Chalmer, T.C. Meta-analysis of randomized controlled trials of cranial electrostimulation. (1995). Efficacy in treating selected psychological and physiological conditions. *Journal of Nervous and Mental Disorders, 183*(7):478-84.

Kosses, R. (2004). Two types of E-Stim. *Rehab Management,* August 2004.

La Fazio, J. (1997). In Vincent, K. Creativity as a healing tool. *Brain Injury Press, 1.*

Mannheimer, J. (1980). *Optimal stimulation sites for TENS electrodes.* San Diego: Medtronic.

Mc Laughlin, C. (1996). Bow-Wow: What a difference animal assistance can make. *ADVANCE for Physical Therapists, 10.*

Medline Plus consumer health information. Clinical trial: Brain electrical stimulation to enhance recovery after stroke. www.clinicaltrials.gov/ct/show/NCT00085657 pp.1-5;

Medline Plus drug information: Lamotrigine. www.nlm.nih.gov/medlineplus/druginfo. 7-05.

Mental Health Source: (1997). New drug helps nerves regenerate. www.mhsource.com from *Nando Times,* March 5, 1997.

Paros, L. & Kirsch, D. (1996). Cranial electrotherapy stimulation (CES): A very safe and effective non-pharmacological treatment for anxiety: A review of the literature. *Medical Scope Monthly. 3*(1):1-26.

Rich, R. (1997). Orthotics and foot dysfunction. Unpublished, written for *Rewiring.*

Robinson, R. (1992). EMD...A breakthrough in therapy. *Bulletin of the Australian Psychological Society.* April 1992.

Schmitt, R., Capo, T., Frazier, H., & Boren, D. (1984). Cranial electrotherapy stimulation of cognitive brain dysfunction in chemical dependence. *Journal of Clinical Psychiatry, 45*(2):60-63.

Seel, R.T., Kreutzer, J.S., Rosenthal, M., Hammond, FM., Corrigan, J.D., & Black, K. (2003). Depression after traumatic brain injury: A National Institute on Disability and Rehabilitation Research Model Systems multicenter investigation. *Arch Phys Med Rehabil.*, *84*(2):177-84.

Schaffer, A. (2007). In latest robotics, new hope for stroke patients. *New York Times*, July 10, 2007.

Shaw, S., Morris, D., & Taub, E. Outcome of upper extremity constraint-induced therapy: Improving function after traumatic brain injury. www.uab.edu/icrc/bireport/6.htm.

Shephard, B. (2000). New strategies after stroke: Restraining, rewiring, relearning. *UAB Magazine*, *20*(1).

Shumway-Cook, A. (2003). *Vestibular rehabilitation.* www.vestibular.org/rehab.html. 2/21/2003

Sivak, M., Hill, C. Henson, D. Butler, B. Silber, S. & Olson, P. (1984). Improved driving performance following perceptual training in persons with brain damage. *Archives of Physical Medicine and Rehabilitation.* *65*:163.

Stahl S. (1996). *Essential psychopharmacology.* London, UK: Cambridge University Press.

Stein, J., Narendran, K., McBean, J., Krebs, K., & Hughes, R. (2007). Electromyography-controlled exoskeletal upper-limb powered orthosis for exercise training after stroke. *American Journal of Physical Medicine and Rehabilitation.* *86*(4):255-261.

Taub, E. & Morris, D.M. (2001). Constraint-induced movement therapy to enhance recovery after stroke. *Current Atheroscler. Reports*, *3*(4):279-86.

Taub, E., Uswatte, G., King, D.K., Morris, D., Crago, J.E., & Chatterjee, A. (2006). A placebo-controlled trial of constraint-induced movement therapy for upper extremity after stroke. *Stroke, 37*:1045-49.

Tufts University Diet & Nutrition Letter. (1994). Shedding dietary light on Seasonal Affective Disorder. *Vol. 12*(1).

UAB Health System. (2003), CI therapy review. p. 1. www.health.uab.edu/show.asp?durk=30491 1/28/2003.

Underhill, A.T., Lobello, S.G., Stroud, T.P., Terry, K.S., Devivo, M.J., & Fine, P.R. (2003). Depression and life satisfaction in patients with traumatic brain injury: A longitudinal study. *Brain Injury, 17*(11):973-82.

Valenti, C. (1998). Panel discussion, BIG meeting, Dec. 13, 1998.

Valenti, C. (1998). Personal communication.

Voelker, R. (1995). Puppy love can be therapeutic, too. *JAMA (Journal of the American Medical Association). 274*(24):1897.

Wilson, C. (1993). Dogs who heal have their day. *USA Today*, 1D, September 21, 1993.

Zasler, N. (1992). Neuromedical diagnosis and management of post-concussive disorders. *Physical Medicine and Rehabilitation: State of the Art Reviews*, 6:33-67.

Chapter Eight: Complementary Therapies

Activator Methods International, Ltd. (2008). Activator methods. www.activator.com/actMethods.asp

Altman, L. (1997). Study on using magnets to treat pain surprises skeptics. *New York Times.* December 9, 1997.

American Chiropractic Association. (2008). The facts are in. www.amerchiro.org/consumer/chi-lbp.htm

AromaWeb. (2008). What is aromatherapy? www.geocities.com/~aromaweb/fwaroma.html.

Bezilla, T. (1997). Traditional osteopathy: Traditional osteopathy as a model for holistic medicine. *The Magazine of the AHMA.* Spring Issue, 1997.

Dannheisser, I. & Edwards, P. (1998). *Homeopathy: An illustrated guide.* Boston: Element Books.

Davids, M. (1997). Alternative medicine. *American Health for Women.* December 1997. pp. 60-63.

Epstein, D. (2002). Network spinal analysis...Introducing the concept of the "spinal gateway." *Chiropractic Journal*, Feb. 2002.

Feely, R. (2008). Cranial osteopathy FAQ. RHEMA Medical Associates Limited www.rhemamed.com/cranfaq.htm

Ferreri, C. (2000). Neural organisation technique. www.positivehealth.com/article-view.php?articleid=585.

Gardner, J.G. (2000). *A healer's voice*. St. Paul, MN: Tree of Life Press.

Horton, C.T. Getting a grip with reflexology. www.doubleclickd.com/reflexology.html.

International Center for Reiki Training, The. www.reiki.org.

Jin Shin Jyutsu, Inc. http://jinshininstitute.com

La Voie, A. (1997). Magnets may help battle depression. Health World Online. *American Journal of Psychiatry*. 154:1752-56.

Lawrence, R. (1998). Controlling chronic pain with magnetic therapy — yes, magnetic therapy. *Bottom Line Health*. September 1998. pp. 9-11.

Lewith, G. Modern acupuncture methods. Health World Online. www.healthy.net/library/books/modacu/mod2.HTM

MacDorman, C. (1996). Acupuncture: America's latest healing miracle: Effective treatment for brain injury. Written for *Rewiring*.

Mahoney, S. (2004). May the force be with you. *Prevention*. October, 2004. pp. 170-171, 200.

Moline, J. Massage is good medicine. www2.spafinders.com/magazine_f_massage.html.

Morter Health System, What's B.E.S.T. for you: The Bio Energetic Synchronization Technique. www.morter.com.

Moyers, B. (1993). *Healing and the mind*. New York: Doubleday.

Naturopathic Medicine Network. What is naturopathic medicine? www.pandamedicine.com/natmed.html

Namikoshi, T. (1981). *The complete book of shiatsu therapy*. Tokyo: Japan Publications, Inc.

Redwood, D. Meditation and relaxation. Health World Online. pp. 1-9 http://205.180.229.2/library/articles/DanRedwood//meditat.htm

Rolf Institute of Structural Integration, The. (2004). Theory and principles of Rolfing. http://www.rolf.org/about.facets.html 9/1/2004

Rondberg, T. (1996). *Chiropractic first*. San Diego: Chiropractic Journal.

Rosenfeld, I. (1998). Acupuncture goes mainstream (almost). *Parade Magazine*. August 16, 1998. pp. 16-18

Rossman, M. What is imagery, and how does it work? Health World Online. www.healthy.net/library/articles/rossman/2imagery.htm

Sacro Occipital Research Society International. Frequently Asked Questions. pp. 1-5. www.sorsi.com/FAQ.html

Tsuei, J. (1996). Scientific evidence in support of acupuncture and meridian theory. *Institute of Electrical and Electronics Engineers, Engineering in Medicine and Biology Magazine, 15*(3).

Upledger, J. (1983). The therapeutic value of the craniosacral system. In *Craniosacral Therapy*. Chicago: Eastland Press.

Weil, A. Healing with magnets? Ask Dr. Weil Q &A. http://cgi.pathfinder.com/drweil/archiveqa/1,2283,149,00

Williams,T. (1996). *The complete illustrated guide to Chinese medicine: A comprehensive system for health and fitness*. Boston: Element.

Chapter Nine: Nutritional Rewiring

Berker, E. (1996). Diagnosis, physiology, pathology and rehabilitation of traumatic brain injuries. *International Journal of Neuroscience, 85*.

Faden, A.I. (1996). Pharmacological treatment of central nervous system trauma. *Pharmacological Toxicology, 78*(1):12.

Gemma, C., Mesches, M.H., Sepesi, B., et al. (2002). Diets enriched in foods with high antioxidant activity reverse age-induced decreases in cerebellar beta-andrenergic function and increases in proinflammatory cytolines. *J Neurosci. 22*:6114-6120.

Mendossa, D. (2002). Revised international table of glycemid index (GI) and glycemic load (GL) Values. www.mendosa.com/gilists.

Morris, M.C., Evan, D.A., Bienias, J.L. (2003). Vitamin E and cognitive decline in older persons. *Arch Neurol.* *59*:1125-1132.

Stein, D., Brailowsky, S, & Will, B. (1995). *Brain repair.* New York: Oxford University Press.

Chapter Ten: Physical Rewiring

Bray, L.J., Carlson, F., Humphrey, R., Mastrelli, J., & Valso, A. (1987). Physical rehabilitation. In Ylvisaker M. & Gobble E. (eds.). *Community re-entry for head injured adults.* Boston: College Hill.

CDC: National Center for Chronic Disease Prevention and Health Promotion. (1996). Physical activity and health: A report of the Surgeon General: Summary. 1996 report, updated 11-99, pp. 1-5.

Dobkin, B.H. (2000). Functional rewiring of brain and spinal cord after injury: The three Rs of neural repair and technological rehabilitation. *Current Opinion in Neurology*; *13*:655-659.

Dordel, H.J. (1989). Intensive mobility training as a means of late rehabilitation after brain injury. *Adapted Physical Activity Quarterly.* *6*:176-187.

Duke University Medical Center. (2004). Long-term benefits of exercise. DukeMedNews. 9/24/2004.

Egoscue, P. & Gittines, R. (1992). *The egoscue method of health through motion,* New York: Harper Collins.

Elrick, H. Exercise — The best prescription. (1996). *The Physician and Sportsmedicine.* *24*(2):1-2.

Engel, F. The Alexander Technique — What is it? www.alexandertechnique.com/articles.engel/ pp. 1-4

Evans, K. (1997). How to gong your own qi. *Health,* March 1997. p. 102.

Gordon, W., Sliwinski, M., Echo, J., McLoughlin, M., Sheerer, M., & Meili, T. (1998). The benefits of exercise in individuals with traumatic brain injury: A retrospective study. *Journal of Head Trauma Rehab.* *13*(4):58-67.

Isenhart, MA. (1992). Personal communication.

Kottke, F.J. (1980). From reflex to skill: The training of coordination. *Archives of Physical Medicine and Rehabilitation,* *61*:551-561

Liu, L. (1997). PulseMind/Body. *American Health, 18*, December 1997.

Mercer, L. & Boch, M. (1983). Residual sensorimotor deficits in the adult head-injured patient. *Physical Therapy.* *63*(12):1988-1991.

Natural Healers. (2004). Hellerwork schools and careers Q & A. http://www.naturalhealers.com/qa/hellerwork.shtml 8/25/2004

Pilates Method Alliance. What is Pilates? www.pilatesmethodsalliance.org/whatis.html

Pilates, Inc. The Pilates Studio. What is the Pilates method of body conditioning? www.pilates-studio.com/docs/method/methwhat.htm

Rinehart, M.A. (1983). Considerations for functional training in adults after head injury. *Physical Therapy* *63*(12):1975-1982.

Rogers, R. (1998). Brain gym helps those on mend from severe neurological disorders. *North County Times,* B-1, 3-Mar-98.

Rosenfeld, A. (1981). Teaching the body how to program the brain is Moshe's "miracle." *Smithsonian,* January 1981.

Smith, A. (1998). Exercise and Alzheimer's: Body & soul. *San Diego Union-Tribune.* Monday, Sept. 7, 1998.

Strickland, B. (1994). How cycling can save your life. *Bicycling,* November 1994, pp. 52-54.

Torp, M.J. (1956). An exercise program for the brain injured. *The Physical Therapy Review, 36*(10):664-699.

Walford, L. (1997). Touched by Feldenkrais. *New Age Journal,* May/June 1997. pp. 51

Wildman, F. (1986). The Feldenkrais method: Clinical applications. *Physical Therapy Forum, V*(8):3-4

Chapter Eleven: Social Rewiring

Albert, S.M., Im, A.; Brenner, L.; Smith, M., Waxman, R. (2002). Effect of a social work liaison program on family caregivers to people with brain injury. *Journal of Head Trauma Rehabilitation, 17*(2):175-89.

Burke W.H. (1997). *Head injury rehabilitation: Developing social skills, Rev. Ed.* HDI Series #9, Houston: HDI Publishers.

Burton, L.A., Leahy, D.M., & Volpe, B. (2003). Traumatic brain injury brief outcome interview. (Abstract) from *Applied Neuropsychol, 10*(3):145-152.

Cicerone, K.D., Mott, T., Azulay, J., & Friel, J.C. (2004). Community integration and satisfaction with functioning after intensive cognitive rehabilitation for traumatic brain injury. *Archives of Physical Medicine and Rehabilitation, 85*(6):943-50.

Elliott, M.L. & Biever, L.S. (1996). Head injury and sexual dysfunction, *Brain Injury 10*:703.

Ergh, T.C., Rapport, L.J., Coleman, R.D., & Hanks, R.A. (2002). Predictors of caregiver and family functioning following traumatic brain injury: Social support moderates caregiver distress. *Journal of Head Trauma Rehabilitation, 17*(2):155-74.

Falconer, J. Substance abuse and brain injury. www.brain-train.com/articles/substanc.htm#Substance Abuse and Brain Injury, pp 1-4.

Feeney, T.J., Ylvisaker, M., Rosen, B.H., & Greene, P. (2001). Community supports for individuals with challenging behavior after brain injury: An analysis of the New York state behavioral resource project. *Journal of Head Trauma Rehabilitation, 16*(1):61-75.

Gosling, J. & Oddy, M. (1999). Rearranged marriages: Marital relationships after head injury. *Brain Injury, 13*(10)785-96.

Grinspun, D. (1987). Teaching families of traumatic brain-injured adults. *Critical Care Nursing Quarterly, 10*(3):61.

Henke, M.E. (2004). Personal communication.

Hibbard, M.R., Cantor, J., Charatz, H., Rosenthal, R., Ashman, T., Gundersen, N., Ireland-Knight, L., Gordon, W., Avner, J., & Gartner, A. (2002). Peer support in the community: Initial findings of a mentoring program for individuals with traumatic brain injury and their families. *Journal of Head Trauma Rehabilitation, 17*(2):112-31.

Hoofien, D., Gilboa, A., Vakil, E., Donovick, P.J. (2001). Traumatic brain injury (TBI) 10-20 years later: A comprehensive outcome study of psychiatric symptomatology, cognitive abilities and psychosocial functioning. *Brain Injury, 15*(3):189-209.

Isenhart, M. (1991). Personal communication.

Jacobs, H.E. (1989). Long-term family intervention. In Ellis D.W. & Christensen A. (Eds.). *Neuropsychological treatment after brain injury.* Boston: Kluwer Academic.

Kautz, D.D. (2007). Hope for love: Practical advice for intimacy and sex after stroke. *Rehabilitation Nursing, 32*(3):95-103.

Kreutzer, J.S., Marwitz, J.H., Hsu, N., Williams, K., Riddick, A. (2007). Marital stability after brain injury: An investigation and analysis. *NeuroRehabilitation, 22*(1):53-9

Leach, L.R., Frank, R.G., Bouman, D.E., & Farmer, J. (1994). Family functioning, social support and depression after traumatic brain injury. *Brain Injury, 8*(7):599-606.

Malia, K., Powell, G., & Torode, S. (1995). Coping and psychosocial function after brain injury. *Brain Injury, 9*(6):607-18.

Perlesz, A., Kinsella, G., & Crowe, S. (2000). Psychological distress and family satisfaction following traumatic brain injury: Injured individuals and their primary, secondary; tertiary careers. *Journal of Head Trauma Rehabilitation, 15*(3):909-29.

Ponsford, J., Olver, J., Ponsford, M., & Nelms, R. (2003). Long-term adjustment of families following traumatic brain injury where comprehensive rehabilitation has been provided. *Brain Injury, 17*(6):453-68.

Powell, J., Heslin, J., & Greenwood, R. (2002). Community-based rehabilitation after severe traumatic brain injury: A randomized controlled trial. *Journal of Neurology, Neurosurgery and Psychiatry, 72*(2):193-202.

Prigatano, G.P. (1995). 1994 Sheldon Berol, MD, senior lectureship: The problem of lost normality after brain injury. *Journal of Head Trauma Rehabilitation, 10*(3):87-95.

Rennell, D.R. (2004). Personal communication.

Sher, J. (1997). My perspective on the family. Written for *Rewiring*. Southern Caregiver Resource Center, San Diego, CA.

Smith, L.M. & Godfrey, H.P.D. (1995). Family support programs and rehabilitation. New York: Plenum.

Wedcliffe, T. & Ross, E. (2001). The psychological effects of traumatic brain injury on the quality of life of a group of spouses/partners. *South African Journal Commun Disorders, 48*:77-99.

Wood R.I. & Rutterford N.A. (2006). Psychosocial adjustment 17 years after severe brain injury. *Journal of Neurosurg Psychiatry, 77*(1):71-3.

Wood, R.L., Yurdakul, L.K. (1997). Change in relationship status following brain injury. *Brain Injury, 1*(7):491.

Ylvisaker, M. (1997). *Management of communication and language deficits. rev. ed.* Houston: HDI Series #20, HDI Publishers.

Ylvisaker, M., and Feeney, T. (2001). What I really want is a girlfriend: Meaningful social interaction after traumatic brain injury. *Brain Injury Source, 5*(3):12-17.

Zasler, N.D., & Horn, L.J. (1990). Rehabilitative management of sexual dysfunction. *Journal of Head Trauma Rehabilitation, 5*(2):14.

Chapter Twelve: Vocational Rewiring

Abrams, S. Social Security Disability Benefits. http://205.188.218.81/sheriabrams/page2/htm.

Asikainen, I., Kaste, M., & Sarna, A. (1996). Patients with traumatic brain injury referred to a rehabilitation and re-employment programme: Social and professional outcome for 508 Finnish patients 5 or more years after injury. *Brain Injury, 10*(12):883-99.

Asikainen, I., Kaste, M., & Sarna, A. (1998). Predicting late outcome for patients with traumatic brain injury referred to a rehabilitation programme: A study of 508 Finnish patients 5 years or more after injury. *Brain Injury, 12*(2):95-107.

Chen, C.L. & Howng, S.L. (1994). The rate and factors of return-to-work in head-injured patients following hospitalization. *Gaoxiong Yi Xue Ke Xue Za Zhi, 10*(6):308-15.

Condeluci, A. (1996). *Interdependence: the route to community.* St. Lucie, FL: CRC Press.

Dolen C. (1991). Use of community services by adult head injury survivors in San Diego County, California. Unpublished Master's thesis.

Farace, E. & Alves, W. (2000). Do women fare worse? A metaanalysis of gender differences in outcome after traumatic brain injury. *Neurosurgical Focus 8*(1).

Haffey, W.J., & Lewis, F.D. (1989). Rehabilitation outcomes following traumatic brain injury. *Physical Medicine and Rehabilitation: State of the Art Reviews, 3*(1):203-218.

Hoofien, D., Gilboa, A., Vakil, E., & Donovick, P. (2001). Traumatic brain injury (TBI) 10-20 years later: A comprehensive outcome study of psychiatric symptomatology, cognitive abilities and psychosocial functioning. *Brain Injury, 15*(3):189-209.

Keyser-Marcus, L.A., Bricout, J.C., Wehman, P., Campbell, L.R., Cifu, D.X., Englander, J., High, W., & Zafonte, R.D. (2002). Acute predictors of return to employment after traumatic brain injury: Aa longitudinal follow-up. *Archives of Physical Medicine and Rehabilitation, 83*(5):635-41

High, W.M., Gordon, W.A., Lehmkuhl, L.D., Newton, C.N., Vandergood, D., Thoi, L., & Courtney, L. (1995). Productivity and service utilization following traumatic brain injury: Results of a survey by the RSA regional TBI centers. *Journal of Head Trauma Rehabilitation, 10*(4):64-80.

Kraus, J., Peek-Asa, C., & McArthur, D. (2000). Effect of gender on outcomes following traumatic brain injury. *Neurosurgical Focus 8*(1).

Malec, J.F., Buffington, A.L., Moessner, A.M., & Degiorgio, L. (2000). A medical/vocational case coordination system for persons with traumatic brain injury: An evaluation of employment outcomes. *Archives of Physical Medicine and Rehabilitation, 81*(8):1007-15.

Malec, J.F. (2001). Impact of comprehensive day treatment on societal participation for persons with acquired brain injury. *Archives of Physical Medicine and Rehabilitation, 82*:885-95.

Malec, J.F. (2005). Personal communication.

Murrey, G.J. & Starzinski, D. (2004). An inpatient neurobehavioural rehabilitation programme for persons with traumatic brain injury: Overview of outcome data for the Minnesota Neurorehabilitation Hospital. *Brain Injury, 18*(6):519-31.

Melamed, S., Groswasser, Z., & Stern, M.J. (1992). Acceptance of disability, work involvement and subjective rehabilitation status of traumatic brain-injured (TBI) patients. *Brain Injury, 6*(3):233-43.

Montgomery, G.K. (1995). A multi-factor account of disability after brain injury: implications for neuropsychological counseling. *Brain Injury, 9*(5):453-69.

National Institute on Disability and Rehabilitation Research Office of Special Education and Rehabilitative Services, Dept. of Education Washington, D.C. (1994). Rehab brief: Community integration of individuals with traumatic brain injury. Bringing research into effective focus, Vol. XVI, No. 8 (1994). ISSN: 0732-2623. www.cais.net/naric/rehab_b/rb-16-8.html.

Oddy, M., Coughlan, T., Tyerman, A., & Jenkins, D. (1985). Social adjustment after closed head injury: A further follow-up seven years after injury. *Journal of Neurology, Neurosurgery, and Psychiatry, 48*:564-8.

Parente, R. & Anderson-Parente, J.K. (1991). Retraining memory: Theory, evaluation, and applications. In Kreutzer, J. & Wehman, P. (eds.), *Community integration following traumatic brain injury*. Baltimore: Brookes Publishing.

Prigatano, G.P. (1987). Neuropsychological deficits, personality variables, and outcome. In Ylvisaker M. & Gobble E. (eds.). *Community re-entry for head injured adults*. Boston: College Hill.

Prigatano, G. (1995). 1994 Sheldon Berrol, MD, senior lectureship: The problem of lost normality after brain injury. *Journal of Head Trauma Rehabilitation, 10*(3):87-95

Ruffalo, C.F., Friedland, J.F., Dawson, D.R., Colantonio, A., & Lindsay, L.H. (1999). Mild traumatic brain injury from motor vehicle accidents: Factors associated with return to work. *Archives of Physical Medicine and Rehabilitation, 80*(4):392-8.

Sbordone, R.J., Liter, J.C., & Pettler-Jennings, P. (1995). Recovery of function following severe traumatic brain injury: A retrospective 10-year follow-up. *Brain Injury, 9*(3):285-99

Sherer, M., Bergloff, P., High, W., & Nick, T.G. (1999). Contribution of functional ratings to prediction of long-term employment outcome after traumatic brain injury. *Brain Injury. 13*(12):973-81.

Social Security Online, The Work Site. Ticket to Work Program questions and answers. pp. 1-5; www.socialsecurity.gov/work/ResourcesToolkit.

Social Security Administration. (1999). Social Security: Supplemental Security Income. SSA Publ. No.05-11000, pp. 1-12.

Social Security Administration. (2001). Social Security: The Ticket to Work and Self-Sufficiency Program. SSA Publication No.05-10061, pp. 1-12

Social Security Online. (2006). The work site. SSDI Employment Supports, pp. 36-42

Social Security Online, The work site. 2005 Red Book. Pg. 1 www.socialsecurity.gov/work/ResourcesToolkit/redbook.html.

US Department of Labor, Office of Disability Employment Policy. Supported employment. (pp. 1-3)

Vander Naalt, J., van Zomeren, A.H., Sluiter, W.J., & Minderhoud, J.M. (1999). One year outcome in mild to moderate head injury: The predictive value of acute injury characteristics related to complaints and return to work. *Journal of Neurology Neurosurgery and Psychiatry, 66*:207-213

Wagner, A., Hammond, F., Sasser, H., & Wiercisiewski, D. (2002). Return to productive activity after traumatic brain injury: Relationship with measures of disability, handicap, and community integration. *Archives of Physical Medicine and Rehabilitation, 83*.

Wehman, P., Sherron, P., Kregel, J., Kreutzer, J., Tran, S., & Cifu, D. (1993). Return to work for persons following severe traumatic brain injury: Supported employment outcomes after five years. *Am Journal Physical Medicine and Rehabilitation, 72*(6):355-63.

Wehman, P., Kregel, J., Keyser-Marcus, L., Sherron-Targett, P., Campbell, L., West, M., & Cifu, D.X. (2003). Supported employment for persons with traumatic brain injury: A preliminary investigation of long-term follow-up costs and program efficiency. *Archives of Physical Medicine and Rehabilitation, 84*(2):192-6.

West, M. (2001). The changing landscape of return to work: Implications for Supplemental Security Income and Social Security Disability Insurance beneficiaries with TBI. *Brain Injury Source, 5*(1):24-27, 48.

West, M.D. (1995). Aspects of the workplace and return to work for persons with brain injury in supported employment. *Brain Injury, 9*(3):301-13.

Index

S

About the Author

Following her brain injury from a 1976 auto accident in a Minnesota snowstorm, Carolyn E. Dolen received the prognosis, "suicide or psych ward." Befitting her feisty personality, she defied that prediction and within twenty years of her trauma earned two master's degrees with high honors, cycled from San Francisco to Santa Barbara in four days and San Diego to Cabo San Lucas in 13 days, and learned to board and kayak surf. Now she defies the concept of "aging" by competing in triathlons and seeking new adventures.

Carolyn's climb up the recovery mountain required rehabilitation in virtually all areas of life, including mental, emotional, physical, vocational, and social domains. (As current friends can attest, she's still working on this last area.) Her *Brain Injury Rewiring* books describe the path others can follow to recover from brain injury.

Carolyn has appeared in print over 100 times, in both authored and edited pieces. Previous publications include columns in the San Diego Brain Injury Foundation newsletter and health/fitness pieces. She also presented at a national ataxia conference and chaired the 1991 San Diego Disability Awareness Week Network (DAWN) activities that received commendation letters and extensive media coverage.

Professionally, she's taught language arts, math, special education, physical education, and health in the Midwest and California to students who range in age from three to forty-three. Currently, Carolyn coaches a stroke survivor at the YMCA and substitutes for teachers in a variety of adult education courses for Ventura Unified School District.

Besides spreading the word about *Brain Injury Rewiring,* Carolyn works to improve her surfing and triathlon skills. She qualified for the 2009 Team USA in the sprint triathlon and plans to place even higher in the future. To balance body, mind, and spirit, Carolyn bicycles, runs, swims, weight-trains, practices yoga, competes in various races, sings with the Master Chorale of Ventura County, greets visitors at St. Paul's Episcopal Church, and volunteers at numerous athletic and performing arts events. Obviously, this rewired survivor doesn't "do" idleness!

You, too, can thrive — "Just Do It!"